HIGH PERFORMANCE HEALTH
TEN STEPS TO MASTERY
WITH PHYSIOLOGY

BOOK 1

Denise E. Plaza and Jill Karlsson Kazikos

ISBN: 148239359X
ISBN 13: 9781482393590

Disclaimer:

This book is intended for informational and educational purposes only. The authors, Denise E. Plaza and Jill Karlsson Kazikos, are health researchers, and Jill Karlsson Kazikos is also a biomedical scientist, holistic nutrition therapist and a specialist in Integrative Functional Medicine. The information in this book is of a general nature and is not meant to replace medical advice. If you choose to use any information presented in this book, it is strongly suggested that you consult with a qualified health practitioner familiar with the subject. If you believe you are in need of medical intervention, we strongly encourage you to seek an evaluation and/or treatment by a medical specialist. The authors (Denise E. Plaza and Jill Karlsson Kazikos) and publication firm (CreateSpace Independent Publishing Platform) shall have neither liability nor responsibility to any person or entity with respect to any damage, loss, consequence or injury arising directly or indirectly from use of information, including recommendations, products and services mentioned in the book.

Library of Congress Control Number: 2013903410
CreateSpace Independent Publishing Platform
North Charleston, South Carolina

TABLE OF CONTENTS

ACKNOWLEDGMENTS

The authors wish to thank the many teachers, scientists, doctors and practitioners of Integrated Functional Medicine who provided guidance, insight and inspiration for this book. Their work is cited frequently because it helped us illuminate both the problems and solutions for achieving superior health. We proudly stand on the shoulders of these people.

We also wish to thank our families for supporting us in our quest to shed light on the invisible and unacknowledged risks of toxicity we encounter in our daily lives and the importance of seeking and sustaining a healthy lifestyle with our behavior, choices, and habits.

Last but not least, we wish to thank our "Team," of colleagues and friends for helping us get this book into publication: Dimitris Michalaros and the design team at KatArt-e, Jane Spurney Michaelides, Janet Kostrevski, Rodica Stavarache, Leighanne Regan, Rick Del Mastro, James Dall and our editors and support teams at CreateSpace.

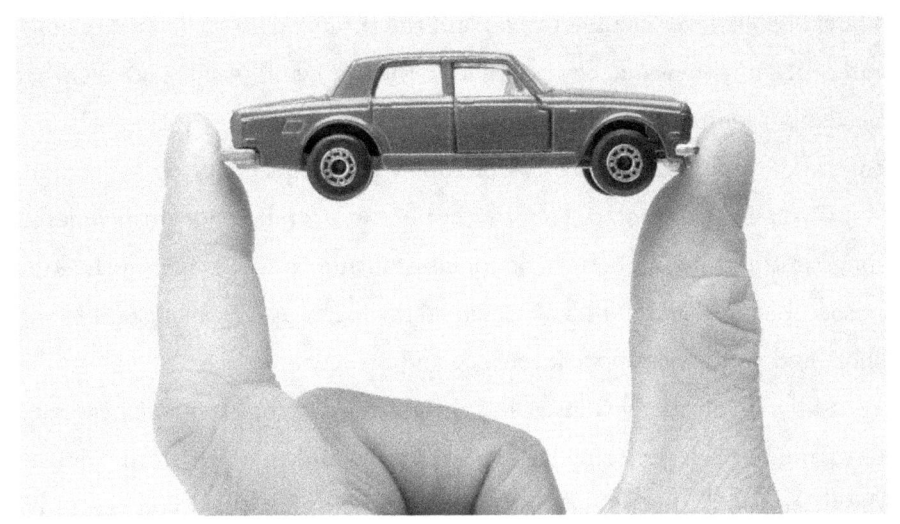

PREFACE:

✧ ✧ ✧

IF YOU WERE A CAR

f *you* were an expensive sports car, would you put low grade fuel in the gas tank? If you owned a world-class race horse that was training for the Triple Crown, would you feed it food contaminated with pesticides and antibiotics or neglect to brush its coat and run it around the track between races?

The answers may seem obvious, but most people treat their cars, and their horses (if you should own one), better than their own bodies. Cars go into the shop for service: you change the oil and filters, you align wheels, and you repair what needs fixing. This could hardly be said about your body. People never change the oil and the filters (assisted detoxification), rarely align it (massage or chiropractic therapy), and usually ignore what needs fixing until they need drastic intervention (hospitals, surgery, doctors, and/or medication to mask or cope with symptoms).

If you want to protect your investment in a car, if you want it to last a long time and be in good shape for commuting to work, taking the kids to soccer games, and not break down on the highway, you bring it into the shop, and you invest in maintenance and prevention.

Sadly, if your body were a car, it might not get the attention necessary to maintain peak performance. The brakes would give out from overuse, the filters would be clogged with dirt and pollutants, and you would be in disastrous shape, mechanically speaking.

If you wonder why you have low energy, insomnia, arthritis, back problems, and chronic conditions like candida, allergies, and migraine headaches, take a serious look at your prevention and maintenance program for your brain and body and ask yourself if you are doing what is necessary to protect the only vehicle you have to carry you through life.

Like an expensive sports car, your body needs the right fuel and the right maintenance to perform at a consistently high level. You not only need the right fuel in the correct amounts, you also need exercise to keep your brain, joints, tendons, and muscles in top gear. You need quality rest, relaxation, and sleep for repair and renewal.

Your ability or inability to achieve or sustain high performance rests on a few key elements, and once you master these elements in your daily routines, your ability to achieve a high-performance life is within your grasp.

These basic elements are fundamental to your well-being and ability to achieve your full potential.

1. High-performance fuel for your brain, the master control center

2. High-quality nutrition for the body to support energy

3. Exercise to increase immunity, function, and circulation, necessary to bring in oxygen and remove toxins

4. Assisted detoxification, the super accelerator for high-performance physiology

5. Sleep, rest, and renewal therapies to maintain balance and focus and reduce stress

6. Confidence, commitment, and attitude

INTRODUCTION:

✩ ✩ ✩

DEFINING HIGH PERFORMANCE (HP)

"The noblest search is the search for excellence."—**Lyndon B. Johnson**

"There isn't a person anywhere who isn't capable of doing more than he thinks he can." —**Henry Ford**

This book is about how to consistently achieve a high level of performance. We give you a simple guide for achieving peak performance in business, academics, research, management, clinical practice, theater, painting, or whatever capacity or professional interest you are pursuing in life.

Our starting point is to define high performance (HP) and the qualities you need to have to achieve it. We state our beliefs and assumptions, so that you know our biases.

Achieving HP is like obtaining a license to fly a plane. We don't sit you in the cockpit, hand you a manual, and say, "Go fly." We would be appalled if pilots were not given the correct amount of instruction and practice flying time. In the same way, we give you the education and guidelines for practicing until you become proficient in the practice of superior health, which is one of the keys to HP.

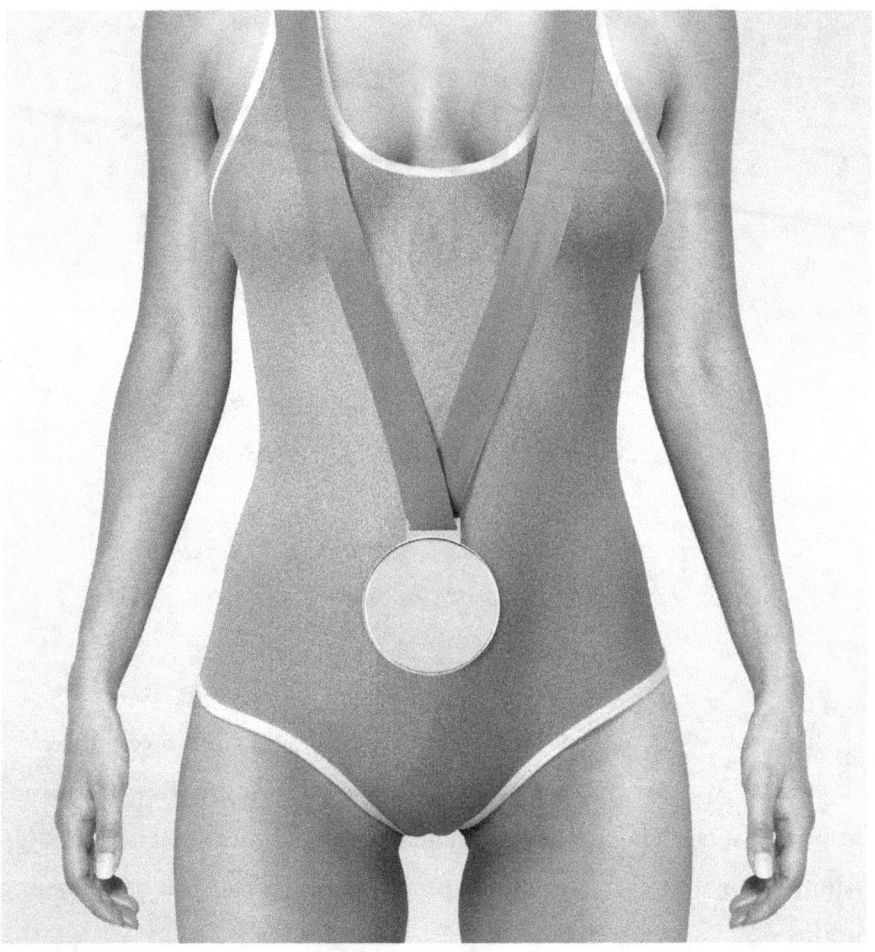

If you search for "high performance" on Google, the entries will be directed either towards athletes or business organizations. If referring to athletes the search reveals what they require to achieve their highest potential, whether winning an Olympic medal, scoring goals, or executing a three-point jump shot. High performance is a strategy to help improve their physical and mental states, which is the basis for their competitive advantage. If referring to business, searches reveal strategies for organization and management, so that they can improve their results. High performance is necessary for both athletes and organizations to become better competitors.

In the same way, for you to achieve your goals, retain your competitive advantage and succeed in business, academia, or sports, you need to implement a few basic principles. Your ability to perform at a consistently high level is linked to two distinct but connected conditions: physiology and psychology.

This book (Book 1) deals with the state of your body and your brain. We start with physiology because once your brain is given the right fuel and your body begins responding to quality nutrition and movement, your path to HP becomes easier, and your focus intensifies. We explain how the body and brain are connected and how to optimize both to achieve high performance.

Psychology is an equally important component, because it deals with your motivation, tenacity, passion, focus and productivity. Book 2 focuses on how to optimize your psychology and your emotional responses.

Let's begin. Look around you. Identify someone you know who is a high performer. If you cannot find a suitable role model, identify someone in an industry you follow or someone on the Internet. One of the most prolific high performers in the "expert" business today is Brendon Burchard. He espouses the basic tenet of this book, which is that high performance requires good health.

You can also look at world business leaders, like David Murdock, the ninety -year-old billionaire who sold his island in Hawaii for $600 million to Larry Ellison, the founder of Oracle. Not only has Murdock been successful in building business empires, but he continues to follow his passions. He built a biotechnology research center in North Carolina, and he actively advances nutrition and longevity. Although most of his loved ones, including his mother, two of his three children, and his third wife Gabrielle, died before reaching the age of 45, Murdoch is optimistic about his chances for living a long life. He is quoted as saying, "I never think about age at all…I just think about what I eat." He believes that the nutrients in fruits, vegetables, seeds and husks hold the key to longevity. Murdoch is still going strong at ninety, and is committed to finding a cure for cancer and finding ways through nutrition and lifestyle to live to 125 years old.

High-profile entertainers, like Madonna, are strict about diet and exercise routines. Gwyneth Paltrow and Jennifer Lopez are vigilant about what they do and don't eat, and they use exercise to maintain their appearance. They don't seem to have problems with weight management, focus, or priorities. Paul McCartney follows a vegetarian diet and, now in his seventies, looks and acts as though he could go on a Beatles tour tomorrow.

A high performer outside the entertainment world is Michelle Obama, whose appearance punctuates her HP lifestyle. Her desire to tackle childhood obesity by improving nutrition and physical fitness is amplified by her commitment to the Healthier US School Challenge (HUSS), an initiative she launched to help schools provide healthier foods in lunchrooms and encourage routine exercise.

Our intention is to make sure that you can identify the qualities and physical appearance that you associate with high performance. Once you have identified a role model, look closely at the characteristics of high performance. You can see that high performers get more things done in less time. They also seem to have good relationships with colleagues, managers, and others in their circle of work and family. They seem to have abundant energy, which is why they are so productive. They are enthusiastic, motivated and, most of the time, annoyingly passionate about their work. They are good at what they do and always seem to want to be better.

We believe that the following qualities define high performers:

1) **High energy.** They can carry a full load of work and more.

2) **Focus.** They give full attention to their projects.

3) **Effectiveness.** They get things done; they are doers.

4) **Productivity.** They juggle many things simultaneously without "dropping the ball."

5) **Stamina.** They hang in there when the going gets tough and the hours are long.

6) **Persuasiveness.** They harness endorsement or approval with convincing arguments and passion.

7) **Passion.** The level of emotional energy invested in their work is positive and high.

8) **Positive mental attitude.** They focus on solutions more than problems and see problems as opportunities and challenges.

9) **Motivation and commitment.** They stay on point to get the job done; they have a perpetual desire to "be better", whether it's better at what they do, better health or better relationships.

10) **Confidence.** They exude certainty about their innate abilities.

11) **Good physical condition.** In most cases, they are physically active and fit.

12) **Strong mental acuity.** Their decision making is well reasoned and accurate.

13) **Balanced relationships.** They have strong, positive relationships.

14) **Discipline.** They develop and stick to routines that support their ability to get things done and maintain physical fitness.

15) **Goal oriented.** They set goals and create a ladder of action steps.

16) **Perpetual learners.** They understand the importance and necessity of education and development.

17) **Role models.** They are natural leaders and usually set an example, which inspires others around them.

Most of these qualities fall into the two dimensions of high performance mentioned: physiology and psychology.

Physiology addresses your physical condition inside and out (your fitness and health). Your physical condition allows you to maintain energy, stamina, focus, and productivity. It can also affect your decision making and mental acuity.

The other characteristics can be attributed to your psychology—the way you think about things. Your mind can determine your attitude, passion, persuasiveness, motivation, commitment, confidence, and to some degree, your relationships.

If these are qualities that you hope to develop and sustain, the guidelines in this book will be useful. If these are qualities that you believe you already have, the question for you is this: Are you a high performer with consistently strong health attributes, or are you a high performer who is successful in many areas but has adverse health issues that get brushed aside because you are so busy?

We want to point out that we have certain perspectives, even biases, that frame our prescription for high performance:

1. A high-performance person needs a high-performance brain. Success starts with the brain; the healthier your brain, the more effective you become at succeeding.

2. "The better your brain works, the better you work."[1] When your brain is fed the right fuel in the right amounts, the smarter decisions you make, the more balanced your Emotional Quotient, Intelligence Quotient, and Lifestyle Quotient (EQ, IQ, and LQ), the better your relationships, and the greater your ability to manage stress.

3. Good nutrition affects your brain as much as poor nutrition. Thinking smart requires eating smart.

4. High-performance physiology, defined by how well your biological systems are working, is essential to high performance. If your biochemistry is not working correctly, neither will you.

Your biochemistry is the interaction of the chemicals that you are exposed to by choice or environmental circumstances. The key biochemical balances are acid to alkaline, blood sugar, and omega 3 to omega 6. The more acidic you are, the more your body is susceptible to degenerative diseases.[2]

5. "Let food be thy medicine and medicine be thy food"— Hippocrates made a good point.

6. The function of your biological systems and the quality of your health are directly linked to nutrition, and nutrition is the key to your body-brain chemistry. You are a chemical and electrical being. The chemical composition of each cell is made and functions with the raw materials from air, water, sunlight, and food. Your electrical being is in each cell; it generates the energy for running your brain and body. Nutrition, the chemicals derived from your food, keeps your body humming (or sputtering, depending on the quality).

7. High performance people make high-performance choices.

8. You are what you think, feel, eat, and absorb.

9. Health is balance. "Health is sustained by a state of balance among countless strands of a web of genetic, physiological, psychological, developmental, and environmental factors."[3]

10. Balance, both biological and emotional, generates qualities that lead to high performance. Balance must be achieved in several areas for the body to sustain optimal health: 1) Energy

expended during the day is balanced by sleep at night, when the body does cellular repair work and detoxification; 2) Stress must be balanced by renewal therapies that restore energy and positive emotional outlook; and 3) Maintain balance with the correct ratio of nutrients (like omega 3 and omega 6 from fish and olive oil, and/or a high intake of vegetables), that in turn yields the correct alkaline to acid ratio necessary for optimal health.

On the emotional and psychological equilibrium scale, we must strive to balance hard work and the hurdles life puts in our path with effective coping mechanisms.

11. "Brain power" and "mind" are not the same, but both require fuel for high performance.

We define the brain as a gray mass weighing less than three pounds. It consists of more than three billion cells and has more than one hundred billion connections between neurons, which conduct the messages in your body. The brain is the control center of your biological, also called autonomic, activities.

The "mind" connects the dots. It helps you decide, "Is this good, bad, or indifferent?" The mind determines how you feel about the information your brain gives you. Your brain is the "keyboard," and your senses "type" the messages. The mind processes the messages and interprets them to create fear, anxiety, happiness, scepticism, joy, and peacefulness (hence the expression "peace of mind," not "peace of brain").

Your mind, your mood, and your feelings are affected by the chemical reactions in your brain (like the release of mood-regulating hormones), which are affected by the quality of your food and beverages.

12. "Most of us are not achieving our full potential for mental health, happiness, alertness and clarity because we are not achieving optimum nutrition for our brain and minds."[4]

13. "A significant proportion of mentally unwell people do not need drugs or do not respond as well as they could to psychotherapy because the primary cause of their problem is neither a lack of drugs, nor a lack of psychological insight or support, but also a chemical imbalance brought on by years of inadequate nutrition and exposure to pollutants and environmental toxins."[5]

14. "At present, medical thinking remains quite linear and simple. Doctors and patients have been trained to think that an illness or chronic condition has a single cause and that it can be treated with a single pill."[6] These authors believe that a holistic assessment is the key to unravelling the causes of illness and disease.

15. "We do not teach in medical schools how to support the natural healing processes." The Western medical model addresses how to mask symptoms with drugs, but we believe that overlooking causes of symptoms can allow conditions to become chronic. Standard medical approaches are geared toward

"crisis health management" instead of health and immunity enhancement.[7]

16. Conventional medicine, while superior and advanced in situations we describe as crisis health, is severely limited in providing best practices for preventing illness. We don't believe doctors are at fault. They are trained to rely on pharmaceutical solutions for problems once they have manifested instead of searching for the cause and helping the patient build immunity; they usually have little or no training in nutrition therapies as potential solutions.

17. An old saying goes like this: "If you want to mop the floor, it is advisable to first turn off the faucet." In contrast to conventional medicine, holistic practitioners of functional medicine (a systems-oriented approach that addresses the whole person and not just the symptoms) are trained to look first for causes. We believe in "turning off the faucet" and determining possible triggers and patterns of behavior that lead to illness. Often this will lead to an assisted detoxification intervention strategy that eliminates what is disturbing the body's system. Detoxification, if done correctly, can "reboot" your biochemistry, re-establish balance, and restart the body's metabolic "machinery."

18. Detoxification is an essential health strategy for high performance. Twenty-first century lifestyles, convenience and food technology have led to an exponential increase in toxic materials, resulting in high levels of toxins in your body and brain. This is catastrophic for the body's detoxification process, re-

quiring that you detoxify so that you can achieve optimal health.

19. Quality, not quantity, defines your nutrient intake. It is not about counting calories but the quality of your macro- and micronutrient intake and your ability to absorb nutrients. No amount of nutrients and calories are valuable unless they can be absorbed and used by the body during metabolism. Although there are many methods to become health conscious, we espouse a methodology that prefers guidelines over restrictions and preferences over dictates, so that you can assess your own bio-individuality and develop your own parameters. You are the best judge of your health.

20. Without commitment and guided change, results and success are not possible. Conversely, if you commit to optimal health and lifestyle changes, enhanced performance will be the outcome.

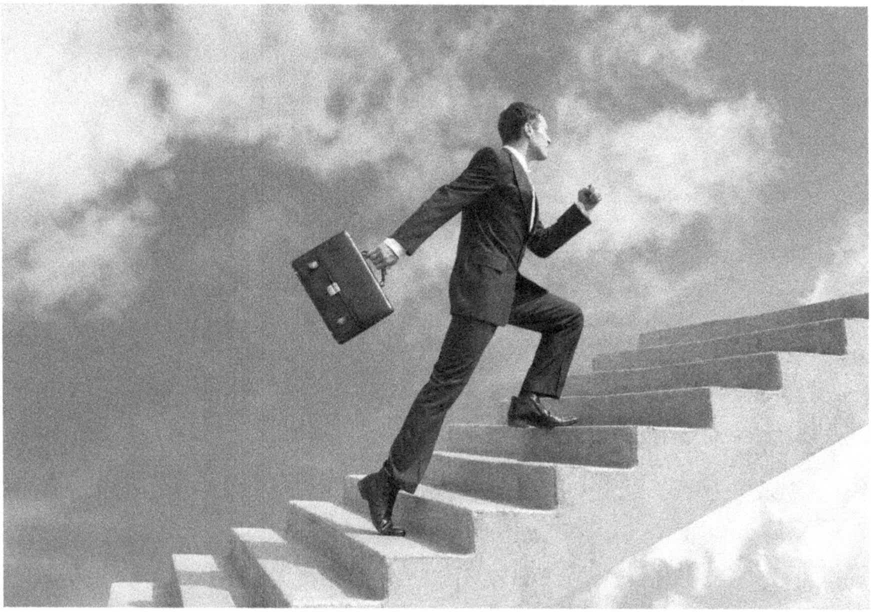

CHAPTER 1:

✡ ✡ ✡

TEN STEPS TO ACHIEVE MASTERY WITH PHYSIOLOGY

"Ah, mastery... what a profoundly satisfying feeling when one finally gets on top of a new set of skills... and then sees the light under the new door those skills can open, even as another door is closing."—***Gail Sheehy***

"Only one who devotes himself to a cause with his whole strength and soul can be a true master. For this reason mastery demands all of a person."—**Albert Einstein**

"Order and simplification are the first steps toward the mastery of a subject."—**Thomas Mann**

We all desire to be the best at what we do. It is one of the keys that can open the door to success, broadly defined as achieving whatever dreams you may have for yourself and your life. However, as one of the best-known authors, Napoleon Hill, in the study of success put it, this concept is not taught in schools. Yet, it is one of the most obvious things to learn in the school of life, because it empowers you to find satisfaction in your abilities and talents and to apply them to the endeavor you decide has the most meaning for you.

Most experts in this field agree that successful people exhibit similar qualities. In writing his famous book, *Think and Grow Rich,* Napoleon Hill studied the habits of five hundred successful people. He concluded that there are seventeen principles that led to success. Two of these principles, Think Accurately and Maintain Good Physical Health, can be summed up in the word "physiology." We focus on your physiology, because it is the starting point for achieving many of the remaining attributes.

These are the ten steps for achieving high performance.

Step 1. Understand that your ability achieve high performance is connected to your level of health. Decide that achieving superior health is a top priority now and for the rest of your life. Once you commit to this goal, make active choices to support this decision.

Step 2. Identify your baseline (current health status) and create simple, attainable goals divided into a specific timeframe for achievement (Action Plan). To attain any goal we set for ourselves, we must first develop a plan. The plan must have deadlines to keep us on track and motivated. Think of it as a journey from one side of a country to the other side. You need a map, where you can clearly identify which roads take you to the other side. Each road will have a number, and you can calculate how many hours you will drive and at which points you will stop and rest.

Your Action Plan will be your map. Once you know where you start the journey (baseline), and where you are going (goals), you can create markers for success.

Step 3. Become conscious of the body-brain connection.

The brain and body communicate as a two-way street. Emotions, stress, and fear can affect your physical body (causing headaches, backaches, and insomnia, to name a few). Likewise, physical exertion and nutrition can affect your brain (making you energetic or tired, anxious or optimistic, motivated or depressed).

For purposes of this book, we are interested in the connection between fuel, the gut, and the ability to function. The gut has more than one hundred million neurons; it is sometimes called "the second brain." This fact is often overlooked or underestimated, but the impact of the gut on the brain is well documented.[8]

Step 4. Start with your head, and work your way down.

The head is the control center of your life; it controls thoughts and feelings, it processes information, it tells you when you are stressed, and it signals danger. It allows you to experience happiness, joy, and the exhilaration of achievement, pride, or a beautiful sunset. If your goal is to a achieve HP and a better life, invest in a better brain. Start with brain fuel, because it impacts the quality of your thoughts and feelings.

Step 5. Learn the basics for superior health or Cellular Energy Optimization (CEO). The fundamental principle of superior health is simple: optimize the performance of the cells in your body, which creates better functioning organs, systems, better balance, and better health. The basic requirements are high-quality water, air, sun, sleep, recharging, fuel, and exercise.

To achieve HP, put more emphasis on the basic fuel and energy supply for your brain and body and be vigilant about removing "energy bandits." These "bandits" can be people who absorb your time and energy. They are also the foods and toxins that deplete energy by using vitamins and minerals to metabolize (sugar) or remove dangerous substances (like mercury in tooth fillings, aluminum, and other heavy metals) without providing nutrients.

Step 6. Exercise daily. Physical activity (respiration and perspiration) generates vitality and energy, builds stamina, and improves brain performance.

Exercise affects the body and brain in numerous positive ways and must be included in any plan to achieve or maintain high performance. Perhaps most importantly, it helps keep the fluids in the blood moving, which brings in oxygen and moves out toxins. If toxins are not removed, they get stuck inside arteries and blood vessels and create conditions for inflammation and degenerative ailments (arthritis, cardiovascular deterioration). Ill health slows you down, detracts from focus, and depletes energy. *High performers know that health and fitness is like an engine; it gives them constant energy so that they stay productive.*

Studies show that people who exercise usually have better performance in a range of cognitive tasks versus non-exercisers. Other studies show that exercise improves longevity.[9]

Step 7. Make choices that maintain balance. Superior health is balance. When you make conscious choices that help your body maintain key biological and psychological balances, your brain function, emotional responses, and health improve dramatically.

Balance, both biological and emotional, generates qualities that lead to high performance. In our prescription for superior health, balance must be achieved in several areas for the body and mind to sustain optimal health:

1) Energy expended during the day is balanced by sleep at night, when the body does cellular repair work and detoxifies.

2) Stress must be balanced by renewal therapies that restore energy and a positive outlook.

3) Biochemical balance is the correct ratio of nutrients, like omega 6 and omega 3 from fish and olive oil, or a high intake of vegetables, that in turn yields the optimal alkaline-to-acid ratio to sustain health.

4) Emotional balance is maintained when you have strong and rewarding relationships with key family members and/or friends.

Step 8. Beware of toxins, and use detoxification methods to assist natural detoxification. Detoxification is no longer an optional health strategy. It is necessary, in your journey for superior health, to become more aware of what can help you nutritionally *and* what can harm you. Toxins can come from the food you eat, the liquids you drink (artificial sweeteners, for example), the dry cleaning chemicals and body lotions absorbed into your skin, the mercury fillings in your teeth, and the fluoride in water. If you lived in the nineteenth or first half of the twentieth century, detoxification as a strategy might not be part of the discussion.

We are exposed to six million pounds of mercury and more than two billion pounds of other toxins each year. The Environmental Working Group (EWG), which uses the power of information to protect public health and the environment, reports that the average newborn baby has 287 known toxins in his or her umbilical cord—a frightening but thought-provoking fact.[10]

Foods are no longer grown on pesticide-free farms but are processed, contaminated, and denatured, leaving them devoid of essential nutrients, and worse, tainted with residual chemicals. Cattle and poultry are not raised to roam or fed grass and seeds (rich in omega 3s, a powerful brain fuel) but are raised commercially and fed antibiotics to keep them from getting sick. Industrially raised animals are not fed grass but soy (which reduces omega 3 and raises the intake of pro-inflammatory omega 6), because it is cheaper.

Step 9. Create your Action Plan, stay committed, and remember that success comes one step at a time. A realistic game plan for improving health should have the eight components explained below.

Each component has an opposite aspect, much as a battery has a negative and positive charge. They represent the balance in your system. Understanding these balances and applying them will help you see the patterns in your daily life.

PHYSIOLOGICAL

In (Nutrition/Toxins)	⟷	Out (Detoxification)
Work, Exercise	⟷	Sleep, Rest, Restore

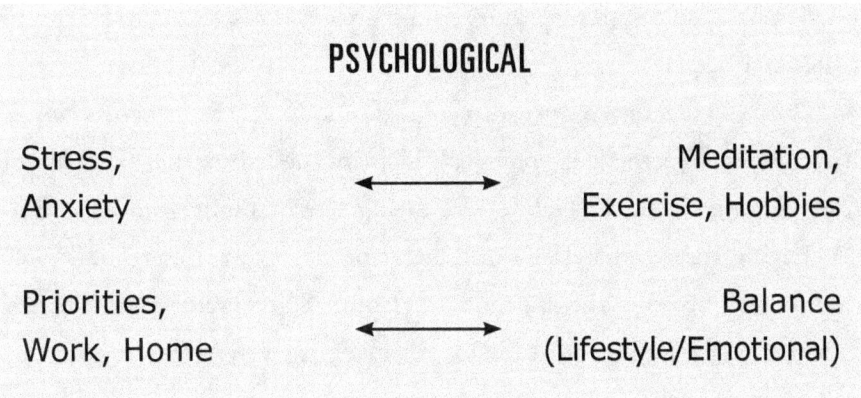

PSYCHOLOGICAL

Stress, Anxiety ←——→ Meditation, Exercise, Hobbies

Priorities, Work, Home ←——→ Balance (Lifestyle/Emotional)

Step 10. Develop new systems and habits. Consciously integrate them into your daily routines to assist you in achieving superior health and a high-performance lifestyle. It is difficult to change habits. You become fond of certain routines; they are like an old pair of slippers that slide on easily and are comfortable, but to achieve high performance, you have to be willing to adopt new approaches.

Our approach is to motivate, compensate, eliminate, balance, and integrate. Begin by defining your journey, setting goals, and identifying personal achievement markers (Action Plan). Once you commit to the goals you set, establish motivation: what excites you and keeps you on track. The next step is to compensate (substitute) for the things you are giving up because they no longer serve your goals. Make positive associations with new choices and less-comfortable routines. Next, eliminate foods, habits and behaviors that do not support you. Last, balance and integrate new habits into your lifestyle until they become second nature.

If you are serious about achieving a high-performance lifestyle, some habits need to be broken, and new habits and routines need to be developed because they support you in your quest for high performance. You need to become a systems creator and manager on the road to becoming a high performer.

Only you can take a mirror to your life and look at your habits closely. If weight management is your goal, identify the habits that prevent you from staying on track. Habits like eating late at night while watching TV, having three beers after work, or eating too many desserts and high-calorie snacks during the day must be eliminated and redirected. We provide you with suggestions to help you invent new systems for your new and improved self.

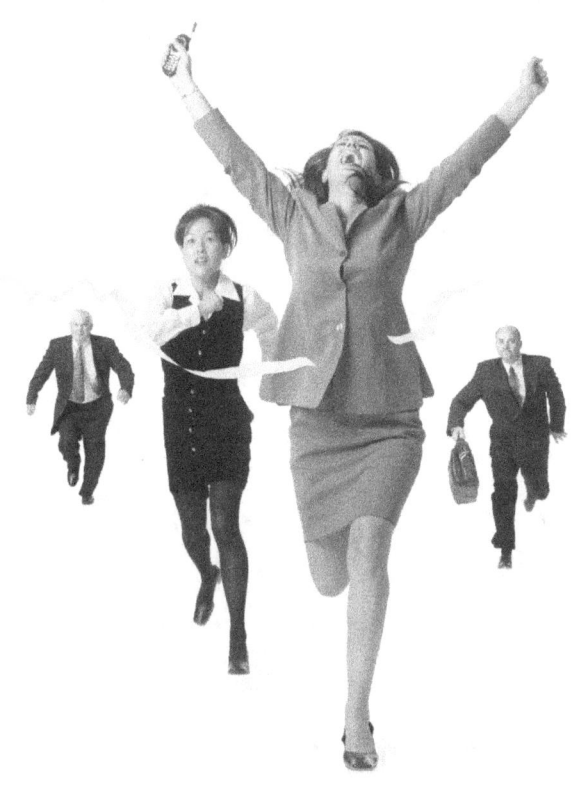

CHAPTER 2:

✦ ✦ ✦

HIGH PERFORMANCE IS CONNECTED TO YOUR LEVEL OF HEALTH

STEP 1: DECIDE THAT HEALTH IS A TOP PRIORITY; MAKE ACTIVE LIFESTYLE CHOICES.

"To keep the body in good health is a duty, otherwise we shall not be able to keep our mind strong and clear." **—Buddha**

*"Without health, life is not life; it is only a state of languor and suffering."***—Francois Rabelais**

"Health is a state of complete physical, mental and social well-being, and not merely the absence of disease or infirmity." **—World Health Organization**

HEALTH IS YOUR COMPETITIVE ADVANTAGE

The decision to maintain good health must remain a top priority if you are to achieve or sustain high performance. Superior health is like a shield and a competitive edge in the world you inhabit. It not only protects you from the diseases of poor diet, lifestyle, and stress (such as heart disease, stroke, and arthritis), it also gives you a competitive advantage. Your brain works better, you are more strategic, you make smarter decisions, and your efficiency increases, so you can stay at the top of your game. With superior health, you obtain one of the most important and defining characteristics of a high performer: energy. The side benefits of energy are stamina and productivity.

Let's go back to the list of qualities we identified as characterizing high performers:

- High energy
- Focus
- Effectiveness
- Productivity
- Stamina
- Persuasiveness
- Passion
- Positive mental attitude
- Motivation and commitment
- Confidence
- Good physical condition
- Strong mental acuity
- Balanced Relationships
- Disciplined
- Goal Oriented
- Learners for life
- Role models

High energy is the first defining quality. High energy can be something you are born with, but it is also a quality that can be enhanced when you are healthy.

What does being healthy mean? This is the critical piece of the high-performance puzzle. The definition we use and the one espoused by the World Health Organization, is as follows: "Health is not just the absence of disease, it is a state of optimal well-being."[11]

We often meet people and ask them how they are. They reply "okay" because they are not sick. Most people believe that if they are not sneezing, coughing, throwing up, or lying in a hospital bed, they are in good health. They even expect to be tired, have headaches, and insomnia, and they consider problems like arthritis the "normal" signs of aging.

The absence of ill health is not good health. This is a false premise, and allows us to accept inferior standards for wellness. The truth, as we have seen in scientific literature and studies on longevity, is that health looks and feels great.

"Optimal health can be defined as experiencing the fullness of life physically, mentally, and spiritually."[12]

Let's look briefly at some of the traits of optimal health, so that you know which qualities to aim for.

Physical Attributes
Youthful and age-defying appearance
Confident and energetic presence
Clear skin
Bright eyes
Shiny hair
Body is strong, usually toned and flexible from routine exercise
Weight is maintained and balanced
Posture is straight and evenly balanced

Physiological Attributes
High energy throughout the day, almost every day
Sleeping patterns are normal, and sleep lasts until the morning
Waking up is not difficult; energy kicks in quickly without stimulants
Digestion is predictably comfortable
Bowel movements are regular, sometimes after every meal
Urination occurs every couple of hours

Illness is rare, and balance returns quickly

Mind is clear and can focus easily

Psychological

Feelings of high energy and exuberance about life occur often

Sexual energy is balanced

Problems and obstacles are seen as challenges; focus is on solutions

Relationships are enjoyable, balanced, meaningful, and satisfying

Sense of purpose is strong

Strong feelings of gratitude and appreciation

The reasons for optimal health as a necessary component for high performance become more obvious when you see the attribute list for health next to the attributes for high performers. It is difficult, and often unrealistic, to expect to be productive, effective, creative, and energetic when your physical energy is not at its optimum level. This is why we emphasize optimal health as your first priority. Begin with this foundational goal, and your other goals will be easier and much more attainable.

HEALTH IMPROVES THE ARC OF YOUR LIFE SPAN (LIFE EXPECTANCY VERSUS MAXIMUM LIFE SPAN)

Dr. Patricia Fitzgerald, in her book, *The Detox Solution,* points out another area measured by conventional health standards that we accept as normal: life expectancy.

Contrary to popular belief, average life expectancy is different from potential "maximum life span." Life expectancy is an average based on how long other human beings have lived, whereas the actual maximum life span possible for humans to achieve genetically is 120 years!

According to Dr. Symeon Rodger, a leading expert on health and longevity, one Chinese man lived beyond 130 years (this was documented by the official yearly birthday wishes he received from the Chinese government).

In researching his book, *Rock Solid Health Qi Gong,* Roger formulated his conclusions about longevity, which he summarizes as "the seven deadly spirals of disease." He postulates that vulnerability to disease is increased or decreased by lifestyle choices, diet, and lack of physical activity, all of which can "spiral" into disease. He says, "Our life style is so sedentary that we lose mobility in our spine and joints leading to injury, affecting the brain and the central nervous system, and eventually to a weakened immune system and disease."[13]

Statistically, fewer people alive today, age seventy, will survive to ninety than was possible sixty years ago. That is because in the early twentieth century, conditions like heart disease, cancer, and Alzheimer's disease were rare. In 1900, one person in thirty-three had cancer, whereas today, one out of three Americans dies of cancer, and one in five develops a cardiovascular condition that interferes with quality of life and life expectancy. The statistics are similar in Europe.

We must not be deceived by statistics that show that the average life expectancy is greater today than it was one hundred years ago. In 1900, the life expectancy at birth in the United States was forty-four years. At the end of the twentieth century, it was seventy-six. The lower number from 1900, however, was due primarily to the deaths of children, because so many of them died due to infection, the result of poor sanitary conditions.

The dramatic increase in survival of children skews the statistics, so when the two statistics are adjusted, taking into account infant mortality, the increase over a one-hundred-year period is 3.7 years.[14]

HEALTH REVERSES YOUR ENERGY DEFICIT TO ENERGY SURPLUS

Poor health takes away focus and reduces overall energy. Instead of using energy for solving problems, being creative, and achieving or sustaining high performance, you redirect your limited energy to fixing your body, because the machinery is sputtering.

If you have a health condition now, you can ignore it or work around it for only so long. Backaches, headaches, or insomnia become worse or chronic. You can take pills to mask the symptoms, but the problem does not go away if you do not look for causes.

In most cases, the causes for health problems rest in a part of your internal machinery that is malfunctioning. When you have superior health, you achieve better balance and vitality in all your internal organs, and many if not all of the problems you were experiencing fade away.

When the "equity" in your "bank of health" improves, you no longer need to rely on deficit withdrawal from the bank, and you no longer need to redirect your time and focus on your body's need for attention. You become freer to live your life the way you choose, and depletion of resources by poor health is limited.

So now that we have highlighted the decision you must make to achieve superior health, the next step is to determine where you stand on the continuum of health.

STEP 2: IDENTIFY YOUR BASELINE AND CREATE GOALS

WHAT IS YOUR HEALTH STATUS?

The only way to get a "license" to fly your health "plane" is to get the proper instruction, followed by the right practice so that flying can become automatic.

First, before we begin, it is important that you establish your baseline health status. The questionnaire that follows will give you some parameters for evaluating your health in four key areas: Diet, toxic load, habits, and stressors. Answer the questions in each category to learn about your health status.

CATEGORY

DIET		POINTS	
	Yes	No	Some times
1. Do you eat 5 servings of fresh fruits/vegetables daily?	10	0	3
2. Do you purchase organic produce/meat/dairy?	10	0	3
3. Do you do most shopping at supermarkets?	0	10	5
4. Do you buy fresh produce in season?	10	0	5
5. Do you eat red meat more than once a week?	0	10	3
6. Do you use sea salt instead of commercial salt?	10	0	3
7. Do you cook with aluminum pots and pans?	0	10	3
8. Do you eat fast foods more than once a week?	0	10	3
9. Do you eat junk food more than twice a week?	0	10	3
10. Do you have frequent food cravings?	0	10	5
11. Do you have a sweet tooth regularly?	0	10	3
12. Do you crave desserts and candies 5+ days/week?	0	10	3
13. Do you drink sodas with artificial sweeteners?	0	10	3
14. Do you buy foods with artificial sweeteners?	0	10	3
15. Do you drink 8+ glasses of water a day?	10	0	5
16. Are sodas/teas/ coffee your main beverages?	0	10	3
17. Do you rely on coffee when you feel low energy?	0	10	3
18. Do you drink alcohol regularly (5x/week or more)?	0	5	3
19. Do you eat in a relaxed environment often?	10	0	5
20. Do you add artificial sweeteners to hot beverages?	0	10	3

Healthy: 130–195

Average: 97–130

Poor: 97 or less

TOXIC LOAD		POINTS	
	Yes	No	Some times
1. Do you smoke cigarettes or cigars?	0	15	3
2. Do you use recreational drugs occasionally?	0	10	3
3. Do you air-out dry cleaned clothes before use?	10	0	3
4. Do you use organic or nontoxic cosmetics?	10	0	3
5. Do you use commercial antiperspirants?	0	10	3
6. Do you wear colognes (men) or perfume?	0	10	3
7. Are you carrying more than 5 kilos (11 lb.) extra?	0	10	3
8. Do you watch TV every day?	0	5	5
9. Do you use an earpiece for your cellphone?	10	0	3
10. Do you swim in chlorinated pools?	0	10	3
11. Do you work/reside in a city?	0	10	3
12. Is your office or house located near a factory?	0	10	3
13. Are you depressed/angry often?	0	10	3
14. Are pesticides used in or near your residence?	0	10	3
15. Are high-voltage power lines near your home?	0	10	3
16. Is your home cleaned with organic/bio products?	10	0	5
17. Do you sleep near a TV that stays on all night?	0	10	5
18. Are fluorescent lights used in your home/office?	0	10	3
19. Are you exposed to second hand smoke 3x/week	0	10	3
20. Do you work near office equipment (e.g., a copier machine)	0	10	3

Low (Healthy): 170–200

Moderate: 99–170

High: 0–99

HABITS	POINTS		
	Yes	No	Some times
1. Do you exercise at least three times a week?	10	0	3
2. Do you consider exercise a priority and adhere to a regular schedule as often as possible?	10	0	5
3. Do you often stay inside all day without breaks?	0	10	3
4. Do you make a point of getting fresh air and sun?	10	0	3
5. Do you watch TV before sleep and in the a.m.?	0	10	3
6. Do you go out of your way to eat healthy?	10	0	3
7. Do you find yourself eating convenience food more than 3x each week?	0	10	3
8. Do you sit in front of your computer for long periods of time daily?	0	10	3
9. Do you use regular detergent (vs. bio) for clothes?	0	10	5
10. Do you have regular routines for releasing stress?	10	0	5
11. Do you meditate 3–5 times a week?	20	0	5
12. Do you smoke?	0	10	3
13. Do you get more than 7 hours of sleep regularly?	10	0	3
14. Do you use coffee/sweets for energy boosts?	0	10	3
15. Do you take walks regularly (3–5 times/week)?	10	0	5
16. Do you socialize regularly?	10	0	5
17. Are your relationships with family comfortable?	10	0	3
18. Are your relationships with friends satisfying?	10	0	3
19. Do you drink 6–8 glasses of pure water daily?	10	0	3
20. Do you relax when you have leisure time (often)?	10	0	3

Excellent: 180–210

Moderate: 90–180

Poor: 90 or less

STRESSORS   POINTS

STRESSORS	Yes	No	Some times
1. Do you feel like you are always rushing?	0	10	3
2. Do you get angry often?	0	10	3
3. Do you accept and approve of yourself?	10	0	3
4. Do you have a strong sense of purpose?	10	0	5
5. Do you find it hard to relax?	0	10	5
6. Do you find yourself judging what others do?	0	10	3
7. Do you have trouble falling asleep?	0	10	3
8. Do you wake up during the night, most nights?	0	10	3
9. Are you in a primary relationship that is nurturing?	10	0	3
10. Is your primary relationship satisfying?	10	0	5
11. Do you dislike your job?	0	10	3
12. Do you feel overworked?	0	10	3
13. Do you feel like a victim most of the time?	0	10	3
14. Do you envy what others have and accomplish?	0	10	3
15. Do you wish you could change jobs?	0	10	3
16. Do you feel that most days are stressful?	0	10	3
17. Is your view of life pessimistic?	0	10	3
18. Do you feel helpless to change yourself and life?	0	10	3
19. Do you become nervous easily?	0	10	3
20. Do you have a hard time making decisions	0	10	3

High stress: 0–85

Moderate stress: 85–170

Low stress: 170–200

The points give you an indication, not a determination. Look at them as a tool to see which areas of your health are strong and which areas and need improvement. If you scored well in each category, you are presumably already functioning at a high level. The information can help you improve your knowledge and strengthen your resolve. Scores in the mid-range show areas for improvement. If you are borderline in some areas, you may need to address poor health patterns, which may require restructuring some lifestyle habits.

Alternatively, you may need to look at work/family balance issues. However, if you scored in the low range in one or more of the areas, take a closer look at those areas, and use the information in these pages to help you address your "weak links." Low-range scores usually indicate substandard health habits and/ or high stress levels associated with poor or deteriorating health, a low level of fitness, poor nutrition, and the beginning of degenerative conditions.

The good news is that no matter what your health status is, there is always room for improvement.

Now that you have an indication of your health baseline, with a view of your weakest link, go back to the list of attributes we identified as characterizing high performers so that you can identify which qualities you would like to attain or improve:

High energy
Focus
Effectiveness
Productivity
Stamina
Persuasiveness
Passion
Positive mental attitude
Motivation and commitment

Confidence

Good physical condition

Strong mental acuity

Balanced relationships

Disciplined

Goal Oriented

Learners for life

Role models

FROM BASELINE TO GOAL SETTING

CREATE A MENTAL PHOTO

Look at this list, write it on a piece of paper, and check the items that are most important to you. Now create a mental picture of what high performance looks like. What would your life look like if you became a high performer? Would you make a better salary, drive a better car, or live in a better house? Would you have more time for your family? Would you look like a million bucks because you are fitter and more confident?

CREATE THE FEELING

Think of how fantastic you feel in your fitter, healthier body, and create the feelings of confidence, exhilaration, happiness, or whatever feelings you imagine in your high performance life. Find a photo that represents these qualities, and put it where you can see every day: on a mirror, on your refrigerator, by your computer screen, or on your desk. This is your motivational "think piece." Think of five things that you will become better at once you achieve your goal. Write them down, and refer to them at least once a day.

Alternatively, think of someone or something that inspires you to become a better you. It could be your child, a mentor, or a thing (a rocket ship, if you aspire to become an astronaut). Perhaps you want to be around long enough to see your grandchildren get married; gather pictures of them. Find an appropriate or representational photo as your motivational piece, and use it as a constant reminder.

GOAL SETTING

Write down five to ten goals that are important for you to achieve (perhaps the reasons that led you to read this book). Look at the characteristics of high performance that you checked, and incorporate them into your list. For example, you might write some of these goals.

1) Improve my energy, stamina, and focus so that I can become a high-powered entrepreneur.

2) Become more productive, persuasive, and effective so that I achieve quality results in my job and get a promotion and a raise.

3) Improve my physical condition by dropping twenty pounds in six months, which will allow me to look and feel better at the next annual sales meeting.

4) Improve my commitment to being more productive by writing and publishing an article in a leading magazine in my industry this year.

5) Learn a new language (or something new or technical).

6) Become more confident and persuasive in client presentations so that I can increase sales by 25 percent this year.

7) Create a better balance of work and home life so that I have more time for my children/grandchildren/hobbies.

8) Acquire (a specific amount of money) for retirement so that I can travel and have enough to enjoy my family without worrying.

Put dates next to each goal, and make sure they are realistic. Losing twenty pounds in a week, for example, is not reasonable, but losing twenty pounds before your annual sales meeting or your daughter's wedding in three months is. If setting a financial goal, see yourself hitting the quota or earning the income through sales by, say, the end of the year.

Put your goal list and the photo of what you will look like in a place where you will see them every day.

Make a mental note every time you look at the photo and the list of qualities: this is what you will look like when you achieve your goal. More importantly, reengage those feelings that go along with the picture, every day.

Every day is a new beginning. If you lose ground, go back to your motivational think piece, and revisit your inspiration.

It is important that your goals remain tangible and inspirational. One doctor, who specialized in learning how the brain works, talked about his goals and motivation. He said that one goal was to live a long, healthy life. His motivation was that he wanted to keep writing and lecturing, but perhaps more motivating than his work was his granddaughter. She was born with a disability, and he believed that being in her life was of great value to her continued progress. He also helped her parents to cope, so he used her picture as the screen saver on his computer.

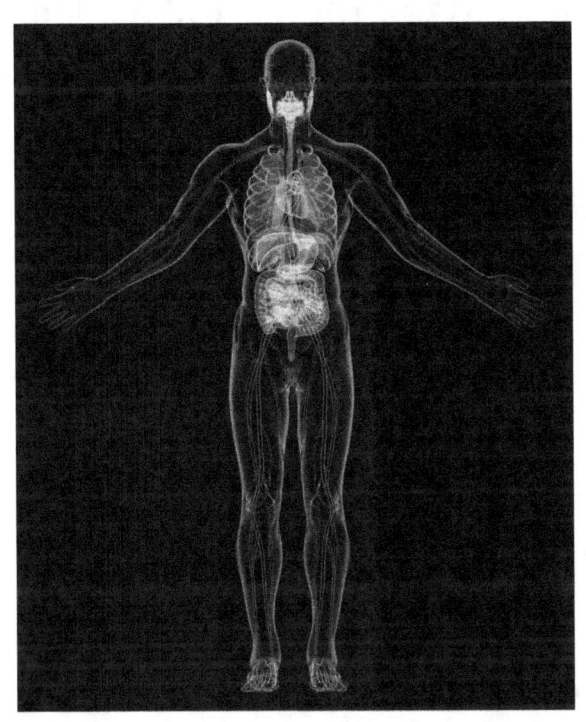

CHAPTER 3:

☆ ☆ ☆

PHYSIOLOGY IS A TWO-WAY STREET

STEP 3: UNDERSTAND THE BODY-BRAIN CONNECTION

"A mounting body of scientific evidence supports the concept that your mind has a very powerful influence on your appearance, your mood, your stress levels, and your overall health. In fact, a whole new branch of alternative medicine has emerged that focuses on the interactions of the mind and body." —**Dr. Daniel Amen**, *Change Your Brain, Change Your Body*

BODY AND BRAIN ARE NOT SEPARATE

"One of the most limiting concepts in the human sciences is the idea that the mind and body are separate. Try asking an anatomist, a psychologist, and a biochemist where the mind begins and the body ends; it is a stupid question, and yet that is exactly what modern science has done by separating psychology from anatomy and physiology."[15]

Anatomically, the brain is a separate entity, encased in a skull, but the mind and body are connected in ways we are just beginning to understand. Once we accept that the entities are not separate, we begin to understand the uniqueness of our biology and psychology.

When emotions and psychological issues rock your world, they often manifest in the body. You may get headaches and feel fatigued. When your anxiety is high, try having a good night's rest. It is generally accepted science that many physical disturbances can be traced to mental or emotional states. Stress is, in fact, the leading culprit and can create a wide range of physical symptoms such as back problems. Medical experts agree that stress is a major contributing factor in chronic illness.[16]

Physicians have long associated psychological stress with cancer. Two thousand years ago, the Greek physician Galen observed that depressed people were particularly prone to illness. In 1846, British medical authorities said that "mental misery, sudden reverses in fortune, and habitual gloominess of temper, constitute the most powerful cause of the disease (cancer)."[17]

Stress slows all the functions that can be "put on hold," such as digestion, tissue repair, and the immune system. The link between psychological factors and the activity of the immune system is now a field of science, called psychoneuroimmunology. This is the study of the connection between psychology, neurological systems, and immune function.

The body is filled with highways of nerves, blood vessels, tendons, and muscles. The skin sends messages when you touch something. Likewise, nerves send signals when you feel an emotion (anger, hurt, or disappointment). The brain processes the input signals and sends a distress signal if the input is negative.

The distress signal can land somewhere in the body and/or it can activate the body's "emergency" system, such as an inflammatory response, that can in turn trigger the growth of tumors.

Consider our five basic states of being: thinking, feeling, action (behavior), energy, and focus. All these states occur across a network of interacting brain cells. We are the sum of all our parts, and each part is intricately connected.

To move, you need a signal from the brain. Actions are a result of your interpretation of sensory input and events, so the brain sends signals across your cellular highways, resulting in your ability to act or behave in a certain way. Even your level of energy is determined by the physical energy in each cell that, in turn, sends signals to the brain.

The senses (touch, smell, taste, hearing, sight) are constantly sending signals from the body to the brain, and the brain interprets and processes each one in an orchestration of responses. Your brain is the master control center. You do not smell, touch, think, act, see, move, or feel without the brain receiving and sending messages.

What is perhaps less understood, or valued, is the effect that nutrition has on mental state. Moods, feelings, memory, focus, and mental energy occur across a network of interconnecting brain cells, and each connection depends on a quality supply of nutrients. Because all conditions start with the brain, the nutrient supply to the brain is the major factor determining how well each function in your body—as well as moods, feelings, the processing of sensory input, and memory—works.

GUT-BRAIN CONNECTION: THE ENTERIC NERVOUS SYSTEM (ENS)

According to Patrick Holford, "How you think and feel is directly affected by what you eat. This idea may seem strange, yet the fact is that eating the right food has been proven to boost your IQ, improve your mood and emotional stability, sharpen your memory, and keep your mind young."[18]

The old paradigm about thinking was that thoughts occurred only in the brain. There are one hundred billion neurons in the brain and more connections than there are trees in the Amazon forest. This paradigm shifted when we discovered one hundred million neurons in the gut, which produces as many neurotransmitters as the brain. This is worth repeating: the gut produces as many neurotransmitters as the brain!

Another important fact about the gut is that it produces two-thirds of the body's serotonin, the neurotransmitter that regulates mood and controls appetite.

What does this mean? Essentially, you feed two "brains." Every time you eat something, the stomach sends a signal to the brain, because your gut and brain are in permanent communication. This is why the right foods make you happy and the wrong foods make you anxious, tired, depressed, or agitated and unable to focus.

With children, the impact of poor food choices is more evident because of their underdeveloped immune systems. Without the correct nutrients, they can become overstimulated, which reduces their ability to focus. This is especially true when children start their day with processed cereal, a high-glycemic* "cereal bar," or white bread with jam or nutella, devoid of quality nutrients and containing an excess of sugar, which then causes the brain to act in weird ways (note the rise in cases of Attention Deficit Disorder [ADD] or Attention Deficit Hyperactivity Disorder [ADHD]). We then wonder why our children cannot focus when they get to school.

The Institute of Optimal Nutrition in London conducted experiments with school children to understand the impact of micronutrients on IQ. It measured the IQ score of school children with a high dose of a megavitamin; a control group received a placebo. The children in the vitamin group saw a staggering increase in nonverbal IQ of more than ten points. Fifteen other studies confirmed that supplements can boost the IQ of children.[19]

Another significant aspect of the second brain relates to the way the neurons communicate with the central nervous system (CNS). Specifically, the brain of the gut, the enteric nervous system (ENS), is involuntary and has sensory neurons that are activated by chemicals in foods. Its one hundred million neurons extend most of the length of the gastrointestinal (GI) tract.

*a food that influences glucose (sugar) levels in the blood

Many of the neurons of what is called the enteric plexuses function independently of the CNS, but they can also communicate with the CNS via sympathetic and parasympathetic neurons, two opposite but balanced biological systems.

The sympathetic system supports exercise and emergencies, also called the "fight or flight response system," and the parasympathetic system supports rest, digestion, and restoration. One increases the heart rate, one calms it.

Emotions such as anger, fear, and anxiety can slow the digestive process, because they stimulate the sympathetic nerves that supply the GI tract.

It is important to highlight that poor intestinal health (lack of adequate and/or quality bacteria in the GI tract due to poor nutrition) can result in these conditions:

Loss of mental clarity (known as "brain fog")
Fatigue
Irritability
Insomnia
Chronic fatigue syndrome
Depression
Anxiety
Mood swings
Back pain
Headaches

As you can see, compromised GI health can create challenges that limit optimal health and high performance.

To better understand the role of the intestines in our health, we need to highlight a few facts. First, the small and large intestines combined measure twenty-six feet and would cover the surface area of a tennis court. Second, our intestines are not just organs of elimination; they are the fuel-use and detoxification control center and have numerous responsibilities that support health:

- They absorb water, minerals, and nutrients.
- They manufacture vitamins like B1, B2, B12, and potassium.
- They break down food residues via beneficial bacteria.
- They form and eliminate unwanted toxic by-products from foods.

Third, the intestines are the key players in our immunity:

- They eliminate poisons, toxins, and waste products that can harm the body.
- They keep disease-causing organisms in check with friendly bacteria.

The intestinal lining is the largest immune organ of the body and it participates in at least 70–80 percent of the immune functions. This is called the gut associated lymphoid tissue (GALT), and it has important implications for staying healthy and avoiding disease. *An estimated one hundred trillion microorganisms, representing more than five hundred different species, including more than one thousand different types of bacteria, inhabit every normal, healthy bowel.* These microorganisms, also called *microflora*, don't make you sick; they are the "good guys." They are the microorganisms that you need to keep the "bad guys" in check.[20]

Our microflora has a multitude of important functions, such as digestion and absorption of foods, synthesis of vitamins, and stimulation of the immune system. Not only does it help you absorb those beneficial antioxidants found in fruits and vegetables, but it also forms a protective lining along the surface of your intestinal tract. The latter then behaves like a vast army of vigilant surveillance soldiers, detecting and protecting us from uninvited microbial invaders.

Research published in the journal *Nutrition in Clinical Practice* also revealed that the microflora in the intestinal tract creates natural controls affecting numerous biological functions in the body, including metabolism, energy production, genetic expression, and nutrition.[21]

This is why you need to keep your intestines in good working order and your gut microflora balanced. A balanced microflora creates a barrier against the environment and prevents the overgrowth of pathogenic bacteria, parasites, etc. Herein lies one of the problems with modern healthcare: the abuse of antibiotics for every ill (although effective only on bacterial infection) has disrupted the gut microflora to the point where most of us need to rehabilitate the "good" flora to get them back in balance. This is because antibiotics are not designed to target only the pathogenic bacteria; they destroy much of the protective, beneficial flora as well.

Other disruptive factors, like pharmaceutical drugs; drinking chlorinated water, sodas, and other carbonated beverages; excessive and/or chronic stress; as well as a diet high in refined sugars and preservatives, can also have a deleterious impact on the good and bad flora in your gut. The result of intestinal imbalance can lead to a myriad of health problems, including but not limited to candida, chronic yeast infections, fungus, issues in the stomach and intestines, depression, and skin problems, as well as food allergies and leaky gut syndrome.[22,23]

Indeed, the rise in health problems can more often than not be linked to the disruption of our microflora.

Conversely, results from more than seven hundred randomized controlled human studies suggest that certain bacteria of the intestinal microflora can *help prevent* diseases from occurring in the GI tract. The studies also show that certain types of bacteria can be used in the treatment of diverse diseases such as inflammatory bowel disease, diabetes, allergies, and premature birth.[24]

When your diet or consumption of antibiotics destroys gut-dwelling bacteria, not only do you lose your main resource for keeping pathogens (harmful microorganisms) in check, you also diminish your immune function and ability to absorb nutrients and digest foods.

The health of the entire body depends on how efficient the intestinal tract absorbs nutrients and eliminates wastes, and since many of the health problems we have today occur because we have disrupted the equilibrium of the gut flora, we need to find ways to rehabilitate our microflora. One good way to remedy this is to take probiotics (means 'pro-life, so guess what "antibiotics" means?).

Probiotics are bacteria that are considered beneficial because they restore unbalanced microflora to a more balanced and healthy state.[25]

So in a nutshell, we have to get the gut to function properly, not only for disease prevention but also because doing so can increase energy, vitality, and positive emotional outlook, all essential attributes of high performance.[26,27]

SYSTEMS THEORY: A UNIFIED BODY SYSTEM

In traditional medical training, a system is a way of dividing the body. Medical doctors are taught eleven specific biological systems and then trained in one specialty. This is why we go to a GI doctor for stomach ache, a cardiologist for heart palpitations, and an endocrinologist for a hormone imbalance.

The term "systems theory" is used in computer technology. It refers to integration, rather than separation. Applying this concept to health, we believe that it is important to view biological systems as unified by their interaction as opposed to anatomical divisions. Functional medicine practitioners look at the whole organism to find disturbances in balance. This is where many unexplained health problems occur—they are not isolated but connected to other systems. A unified approach allows a practitioner to assess balance among multiple systems, and balance is one of the most important keys in our formula high-performance health.

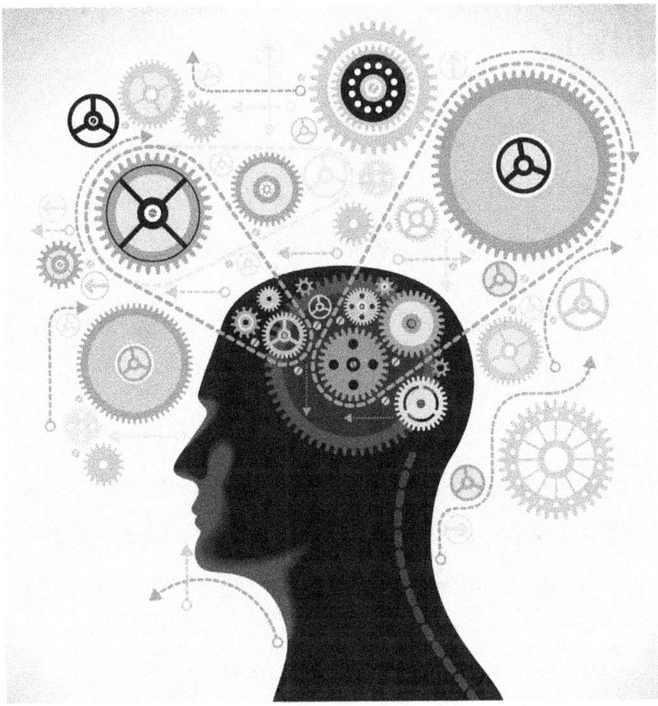

CHAPTER 4:

✡ ✡ ✡

HIGH PERFORMANCE STARTS IN YOUR BRAIN

STEP 4: START WITH YOUR HEAD AND WORK YOUR WAY DOWN.

"I am a brain, Watson. The rest of me is a mere appendix."
—**Arthur Conan Doyle**, *The Adventure of the Mazarin Stone*

CONTROL CENTRAL: THE MAGNIFICENT BRAIN

"Brains run the world." As Dr. Daniel Amen, one of the leading experts in brain health describes it, "Brains run the stock market, the local market, huge corporations, and the mom and pop shops down the streets...governments, schools, churches, families, organizations, and you." According to Amen, "Brain Excellence is your competitive advantage in ANYTHING that you do, because success ALWAYS starts with a healthy brain."[28]

We couldn't agree more. The healthier your brain, the better the quality of your thinking. The quality of your decision making is directly related to and a function of the health of your brain, so if you want to become a high-performance person, start with your brain.

According to Patrick Holford, a renowned British nutritional therapist, "most of us are not achieving our full potential for mental health, happiness, alertness and clarity because we are not achieving optimum nutrition for the mind."[29]

The brain is unlike any other organ: it weighs less than 3 lb. (1 1/2 kilos), is composed mostly of water and fat, and has the consistency of something between Jell-O and oatmeal. It is encased in a hard, bony structure called our skull, and it controls every thought, mood, impulse and reaction we have, whether conscious, or unconscious. Three pounds of your body mass controls how you think, act, behave, get along with people, perceive beauty, pain, happiness, and joy, make decisions, plan a party or plan your life. It is your character, your personality, and your judgment. Everything starts with your brain.

Recall that we make the distinction between your brain, which takes raw data and gives you feedback so that you can recognize a friend or the sound of a bird versus a dog, and your mind. The mind interprets the data it receives.

This is the reason to start the journey to HP with a decision to seek health and a commitment to make changes that support your decision. Deciding is the starting point for any goal, and it starts in your brain, with a kick from your mind. Make sure your mind is on board if you desire to succeed.

HOW THE BRAIN WORKS

The brain operates by conducting signals through a vast network of neurons with special nerve cells that connect to other neurons. It is impossible to fathom how many neurons we have: think of every phone connection in the world, including mobile phones, and you are still short by two billion connections. The brain conducts signals between one hundred billion neurons—that is more than the stars in the universe! (There are ten billion stars in the Milky Way.)

Neurons do not touch, and the connections between them, dendrites, have a gap between them called synapses. All the signals and messages about what you think, feel, touch, see, or hear is carried from one neuron to another across the gap, like the action of a spark plug in a car.

The messages are sent and received from stations on each neuron, and these stations are built from fats—not any fats, but fats that the body cannot manufacture. They must be obtained from food you eat, which is why they are called "essential fats." The fats you consume be-come the construction material that your brain uses to send and retrieve messages.

SMART FATS BOOST YOUR INTELLIGENCE

"Conclusive research now clearly shows that the amount and type of fat consumed during fetal development, infancy, childhood, adolescence, adulthood, old age-indeed every day of your life-has a profound effect on how you think and feel. The brain and nervous system are totally depen-dent on a family of fats."[30]

The smart fats, the essential fatty acids, are the omega 3s and omega 6s. Saturated and monounsaturated fat, cholesterol, and phospholipids are important, but these can be made in the body. Omega 3 and 6 must be obtained from diet, hence, they are essential.

This means that if the food you eat does not include the right amount of these essential fats, your brain is not getting them. Period. If your brain is not getting them, your ability to be healthy and to have a high-performance brain is compromised.

The smart fats are critical for mental health. They not only stave off deteriorating conditions from depression, fatigue, and memory loss to Alzheimer's disease and schizophrenia, but they also reduce the risk of cancer, heart disease, allergies, arthritis, eczema, and infection.[31]

In optimal amounts, they are indispensable if you want to maximize brain performance. All the deteriorating brain conditions just mentioned have been linked to deficiencies of omega 3. Conversely, the correct amount of omega 3 fats, balanced with omega 6, can have a tremendous impact on how you function emotionally (stress and anger control), physi-cally (coordination), and intellectually (choices, reasoning, conceptualiza-tion, and innovation).

Studies show that animals with low essential fats perform poorly on mental intelligence tasks and show poor memory. Similar studies with children show that learning difficulties are associated with low levels of essential fats.

MORE EVIDENCE

Donald Rudin, a doctor and medical researcher, conducted research showing that flax oil improves the behavior of schizophrenics and juvenile delinquents who fail to respond to counselling. An ongoing research program at Hammersmith Hospital in London demonstrated that babies of vegan mothers who breastfed were brainier. The link appears to be that the breast milk of dairy-eating vegetarians provided more of the essential fatty acids needed for the development of neural membranes.[32]

The omega 3 and omega 6 fats are obtained from salmon, fish oil, sardines, cod, and some nuts like walnuts.

Brain cells communicate with one another instantaneously, sending and receiving messages via synapses, without touching. Every receptor site is contained in a myelin sheath, which is like the insulation around electrical wiring. This electrical wire is roughly 75 percent fat, and its insulation is made out of phospholipids, another important nutrient in the arsenal of smart fats.

Phospholipids are the insulation for your brain "wiring." They make the myelin sheath around the nerves, which allows the signals to communicate smoothly. The deterioration of this lining is responsible for degenerative brain conditions like Parkinson's disease, Alzheimer's disease, and multiple sclerosis. All these diseases occur because of poor nerve communication. The signals can no longer fire across the synapses as they used to because the nerve sheaths are destroyed.

DEBUNKING THE BAD EGG MYTH

The richest sources of phospholipids are egg yolks, organ meats, and lecithin derived from plant sources, which is why the king of the animal world, the lion, stays on top of the food chain. He eats the organs and brain of his prey first.

In Chinese medicine, eggs are considered one of the perfect foods. They are the richest source of choline, which is responsible for acetylcholine, the memory neurotransmitter. Deficiency in choline is the most common cause of memory decline, but the quality of the egg depends on the chicken's diet. If the chicken is fed flaxseeds and fishmeal, for example, the eggs will be rich in omega 3 and phospholipids. When buying eggs, check your source (organic or omega 3 eggs are best).

Fears about eggs raising cholesterol are misguided, because they are based on a partial understanding of why we have high cholesterol. The body not only produces cholesterol, it requires it. Your brain contains huge amounts of it, and it is essential for manufacturing sex hormones like estrogen, progesterone, and testosterone. For people who wish to lower their cholesterol, it is often good to start by looking at an entire eating and lifestyle program, including the amount of daily exercise (which significantly reduces bad cholesterol). A holistic evaluation will identify the real culprits for cholesterol problems. Diets rich in red meat, refined flour and sugar, bad fats like cream and fried foods, and lack of exercise are the likely source of cholesterol problems, not eating eggs.

AMINO ACIDS: LETTERS FOR THE BRAIN'S MESSAGES

The macronutrients in the "smart brain" landscape are proteins, which are made from amino acids.

The messages that the brain sends between the stations are called neurotransmitters, and these are made of amino acids derived from proteins. The neurotransmitters are chemical messengers that neurons use to communicate impulses: some trigger an impulse telling neurons to receive an impulse, and others trigger an impulse to stop neurons from retrieving one. They are used like postal letters, or "text messages," from one cell to another.[33]

Different amino acids make different neurotransmitters. For example, dopamine, which helps you feel buoyant and happy, is made from the amino acid phenylalanine (and tyrosine). Adrenaline and dopamine are the hormones that keep you motivated, and they are made from the amino acid phenylalanine. Neurotransmitters are made directly from amino acids taken into the body from food. Just as certain fats are essential because the body can't make them, there are eight essential amino acids that you should eat so that you can make the important neurotransmitters.

To make sure you are getting your essential amino acids, eat at least two servings of protein-rich foods every day. Good-quality vegetable protein sources include lentils, quinoa, tofu, beans, and seed vegetables. If you prefer meat, stick to lean cuts, fish, and poultry. Buy organic whenever possible to reduce the amount of toxins you ingest with food.

In addition to dopamine, the happy mood neurotransmitter, and adrenaline, the motivation neurotransmitter, there is tyrosine, which is critical to mental and physical performance, especially under stressful circumstances. This was recently confirmed by research conducted by the US military. "Studies by the U.S. military found that giving tyrosine to soldiers in stressful conditions of extreme cold, or intense physical activity over prolonged periods of time show clear improvements in both mental and physical endurance."[34]

If you are stressed, serotonin (mood-regulating, stress-lowering neurotransmitter) and tryptophan calm you and help you sleep better.

We know that the brain needs high-quality essential fats to support the synapses, the messages, and the send-and-receive stations. It needs certain essential amino acids to support mood, increase mental acuity and physical abilities, and stimulate motivation.

If you are now asking yourself, "How do I get more of the motivation and happy neurotransmitters?" you need another piece of the puzzle. To make the neurotransmitters out of amino acids, the body depends on enzymes in the brain, and these enzymes require the right kind of micronutrients found in vitamins and minerals.

MICRONUTRIENTS: MASTER CONTROL LEVERS FOR THE BRAIN

During every movie or show, there are the actors on the stage, the people who get the spotlight, and the people "behind the scenes," the worker bees, who make sure that every scene has the right lighting and the furniture is in the right place. If your brain puts on a show every day, the behind-the-scenes support staff members are the micronutrients: the vitamins, minerals, and phytochemicals that fine-tune every performance.

One of their main roles is to turn glucose into energy, amino acids into neurotransmitters, simple essential fats into more complex fats like gamma-linolenic acid (GLA), docosahexaenoic acid (DHA), and prostaglandins, and choline and serine into phospholipids, the insulation for the brain wiring.[35]

The body uses micronutrients to rebuild cells, create energy, and insulate the body, as well as protect it from harmful substances.

Vitamins and minerals are so crucial to health that a study commissioned by the Council for Responsible Nutrition in America estimated that $8.7 billion could be saved annually from reduced hospitalizations resulting from the five major diseases (heart disease, cancer, stroke, lung disease, and diabetes) if the foods consumed contained the antioxidant vitamins A, C, and E. The $8.7 billion figure implied a five-year savings of more than $43.5 billion. [36]

Furthermore, according to a review of nutrition initiatives directed toward disease prevention, "it has been predicted that healthier dietary practices could save $71 billion per year in medical costs, lost productivity, and the value of lives lost prematurely to heart disease, cancer, stroke and diabetes." [37]

Most people eat fewer than one or two portions of fruits and vegetables each day. This is in stark contrast to what the Recommended Dietary Allowances (RDA), the Institutes for Health, and many nutritionists believe is the optimal, health promoting amount (at least five portions).

Joel Fuhrman, an American board-certified physician who specializes in nutrition-based treatments for obesity and chronic disease, said, "Micronutrient-poor foods, like pasta, sugar, and soda, don't just give you empty calories and make you fat, they also do damage to the body and cause disease." He also says, "Without micronutrients to remove waste, cells become congested. DNA gets broken, and the body doesn't have the ability to repair itself. Eventually you get sick."[38]

Fuhrman developed what he calls a "nutri-tarian diet" of foods with the most micronutrients per calorie. Because most micronutrients aren't listed on labels, he created a thousand-point Aggregate Nutrient Density Index (ANDI), which ranks foods based on micronutrient concentration.

In his index, leafy green vegetables dominate the upper end of the ANDI, scoring between 500 and 1,000, while radishes, cabbage, and broccoli score in the 300 to 500 range. Fruit averages 100, and nuts and seeds are between 17 and 124. Not surprising, meat and dairy fall at the bottom range (2 to 39).

According to Manuel Villacorta, a spokesman for the American Dietetic Association, "Eating these (micronutrient rich) foods is great for cardiovascular health and fighting high blood pressure and cancer…in every bite, you get hundreds of antioxidants and anti-inflammatories."[39]

Scientists are beginning to appreciate the importance of these nutrients, and we could write volumes on the impact of these "worker bees" on thinking and health. Every one of the fifty known essential nutrients plays a major role in promoting mental acuity.[40] To illuminate their importance, we are highlighting just a few:

B-COMPLEX VITAMINS: A BOOST FOR BRAIN FUNCTION

The B-complex group of vitamins—B1 (thiamine), B3 (niacin), B5 (pantothenic acid), B6, B9, B12, folic acid, biotin, and choline—are critical to the functions of the brain like memory and how you feel. Signs of deficiency in these vitamins include memory loss, poor concentration, impaired learning, and general forgetfulness. Most importantly, B-complex vitamins are essential for the production of cellular energy, particularly in brain cells, so make a note of how you can improve your mental performance with these foods. Good sources include chicken, collards, kale, oatmeal, soy beans, fish, avocados, brewer's yeast, turkey, halibut, nuts and seeds, apricots, leafy green vegetables, and whole grains.

Vitamin B1 helps turn glucose into energy, so if you become deficient in B1, you experience mental and physical tiredness. People with low vitamin B1 also have poor attention spans and concentration.

Vitamin B3 (niacin) deficiency is found to cause pellagra, a disease where people develop mental illness, diarrhea, and eczema. Correct levels, in contrast, can improve memory in young and old people by as much as 10 percent.

Vitamin B5 (pantothenic acid) is a potent memory booster that is needed to make stress hormones and the memory-boosting neurotransmitter, acetylcholine.

The B6, B12, and folic acid group, together with niacin, plays a critical role in the body's ability to make almost all the neurotransmitters.

Without B12, the brain and the senses cannot work properly. Deficiency shows up in people with dementia.

Choline is transformed into acetylcholine, a neurotransmitter responsible for sending information from one brain cell to the next. Low levels of acetylcholine cause memory loss in varying degrees from "it's on the tip of my tongue" to complete lapses.

OTHER BRAIN HELPERS

Vitamin C helps balance neurotransmitters; studies show that it helps reduce symptoms of depression and schizophrenia. Sources include citrus fruits, red bell peppers, dark leafy greens, and broccoli.

Calcium and magnesium relax nerve and muscle cells, and they work together, so anxiety and nervousness can often be helped by this duo. You can find calcium in dairy products like yoghurt, but keep in mind that broccoli also provides ample calcium, enough for healthy menstrual cycles and normal blood pressure.

Magnesium, one of the most common mineral deficiencies, plays an important role in the nervous system and has been linked to mental illness. The best sources include green leafy vegetables, nuts, and seeds, like sesame, sunflower, and pumpkin.

There are many other micronutrients that help brain cells function better, but if you stick to the rule that "more is better when it comes to veggies" and eat a minimum of five servings a day, you will kick start your brain function.

BRAINS ARE HOGS

The brain is a "hog" when it comes to energy consumption. Even though it weighs less than three pounds, it consumes almost 60 percent of the glucose energy of the entire body. Three pounds is probably less than 2 percent of your body mass (if you weigh between 135 and 150 pounds), so 2 percent of your body is using 60 percent of your energy! It is clearly the most expensive "real estate" in your body. When you think about what your brain accomplishes every day, in conscious and non-conscious moments, it is not surprising.

It processes every sensory input, and gives instructions to your organs, muscles, eyes, ears, digestion, kidneys, telling them what to do and when and how to do it. Even when you sleep, your brain is in charge of sanitation and clean-up. Most of the body's detoxification, which is essential for health and requires a great deal of energy, occurs while you sleep.

The neurons are sending and receiving stations for all information, and with ten trillion cells communicating with one another every second, it has a lot of management responsibility. Nevertheless, we hardly think about what the brain needs in order to function at a high level.

HIGH OCTANE GLUCOSE: SMOKELESS FUEL FOR SMART BRAINS

The best fuel for the brain comes from complex carbohydrates, which are whole grains, vegetables, beans, and lentils. Some fruits, although they are simple carbohydrates, can also be good fuel, because they take longer to digest than refined carbohydrates.

You may be asking, "What is it about complex carbohydrates that make them the best fuel for my body?" The answer is that they are digested differently, and when broken down into the necessary fuel, glucose, they do not leave a residue of toxins that the body must dispose of. Glucose can go right to the brain.

You make energy from proteins, fat, and carbohydrates. The complex carbohydrate varieties are not only a "smokeless" fuel, they are slow releasing. Energy is released slowly and gradually, which helps keep your blood sugar balanced.

WRAP YOUR HEAD AROUND THIS THOUGHT: YOU THINK WHAT YOU EAT AND ABSORB

We know that the composition of the brain is water and fat. We know that the composition of brain messages is amino acids from proteins, and we know that the top-notch fuel supply is glucose from complex carbohydrates.

We also know that the brain operates by sending messages (neurotransmitters) between sending-receiving stations (neurons), which are composed of fats. The quality of the transmissions, over six thousand thoughts a day, depends on the quality of the sending-receiving stations and the ability of the cells to communicate effectively.

If the brain is mostly water and fat, and these molecules control our wiring, amino acids are the raw materials for the messages, and glucose is the fuel, then it would make sense that we should supply the brain with these nutrients. More importantly, they should be of the highest quality, because this impacts our thinking.

Our current health paradigm may have a few things upside down. For example, we are told to keep away from fats because they can clog our arteries and spike our cholesterol. However, we are not told that there are two types of fat in food. One helps manufacture hormones, including sex hormones, keeps our cell membranes fluid and permeable, and contributes to the brain's ability to function at a high level. The more dangerous type we get from fried foods, processed foods, trans fats, and excess quantities of saturated fat found in animal meats; these can cause elevated cholesterol, clogged arteries, and poor health.

One of the most important facts you will learn from this book is that food is made of "good guys" and "bad guys." Hippocrates is quoted as saying, "Let food be thy medicine, and medicine be thy food," but Hippocrates could not have anticipated the toxic overload of the twenty-first century. If he had had a crystal ball, he would have warned, "Beware of foods that can be your poison, for they will cause disease, damage your musculoskeletal system, and make you fat."

GOOD GUYS, BAD GUYS

The food supply has "good" carbs and "bad" carbs, good fats and bad fats, foods that give you energy and foods that rob you of energy. The tricky part is to get a handle on these distinctions so that you can start flying your health "plane" to high performance.

Fats are metabolized differently from other nutrients. The significance of this is that your brain is literally made from the fats you eat. Eat rancid fats (such as French fries that are repeatedly fried in the same oil in fast food restaurants), and your cell membranes (or should we say *membrains*) become more permeable. Eat high-quality fats, and your brain synapses act like a spectacular display of fireworks. They can shoot messages back and forth, and the quality of transmission is high and fast. Think of the first computer you owned and its speed versus the newer models. Your brain can be like a computer with "old memory" or a high-speed, large-memory computer just by changing the materials it uses to create its neuro-highways.

Although you need to balance fats, the good fats are primarily mono-unsaturated and polyunsaturated. How do you know which is which? When a fat is liquid at room temperature, it is mono or polyunsaturated. When it is hard at room temperature, it is saturated.

Studies have shown correlations between poor heart health and heavy quantities of saturated fats from animal meats. The US Department of Agriculture (USDA) and the American Heart Association (AHA) recommend that saturated fats represent less than 7 percent of your fat intake.[41] We believe that it is not saturated fats per se that are detrimental to health but rather the balance of good fats to bad fats and the combination of exercise and other lifestyle factors. To ensure you get the proper balance however, just remember to favor liquid (monounsaturated oils), instead of hard (saturated fats) in your diet.

WHITE IS YOUR ENEMY, COLOR IS YOUR ALLY

What about carbohydrates? Just like fats, there are differences in the quality of carbohydrates. Most of the white carbohydrates in a modern diet are low-grade fuel for the brain. The "white enemy" is easy to identify because it's white: white rice, white sugar, white pasta, white bread, white crackers, white cake, and white cookies. All of these products are made with refined sugar and refined flour. If you want to know why your blood sugar is unbalanced, why you have mood swings, why your energy is low, or why you can't seem to lose weight, look your enemy in the eye. It is in your cupboard and on your food plate. It is white.

In contrast, all your strong health allies are full of color. All the good carbs come from fruits, vegetables, whole grains, and legumes. If you cannot remember this list, think color and avoid white. The more colorful the fruit or vegetable is, the higher the nutrient value. Rule number one for better health is to enrich your diet with color: red peppers, broccoli, kale, spinach, and apples. Look for green, red, purple, orange, and even indigo and blue. Think blueberries, plums, and eggplant. There are some notable exceptions in the white department (like mushrooms and some eggplant varieties), and we are not asking you to avoid these because they are part of the vegetable family.

Build your smart food repertoire so that you can discriminate good carbs from empty, fat-enhancing, bad carbs.

Another tool for identifying a good carb is to determine how many ingredients it has. To be high quality, it should have one ingredient—if you want to rid yourself of bad carbs, think of the one-ingredient rule. Apples, pears, strawberries, tomatoes, avocados, arugula, spinach, broccoli, and sweet potato are all one ingredient. The closer you get to this standard, and the more abundant your diet is with fruits and vegetables, the closer you are to superior health and an HP brain.

Think about what you buy in the supermarket. How many packaged foods do you buy and put in your pantry or refrigerator? How many snacks do you eat during the day? Do they come in a package? Look at the number of ingredients listed. These are what we consider the "bad carbs", and they also have bad fats. If you check the ingredient list and it includes partially hydrogenated or hydrogenated oil, you are consuming trans fats, one of the most insidious toxins in your diet.

Packaged foods should be avoided, because they are loaded with artificial ingredients and coloring, and they contain bad fats, trans fats in particular. They are also generally poor in quality nutrient carbohydrate value.

"Sugars and stimulants make you stupid." Patrick Holford, Optimum Nutrition for the Mind

In *Optimum Nutrition for the Mind*, brain expert Patrick Holford characterizes sugar as the worst fuel for the brain: the kind you find in most packages on a supermarket shelf, boxed cereal, cookies, cakes, crackers, and all the "white" enemies. It is also the kind of sugar found in the candy bars, snack bars, granola bars that children like to get after school.

Refined carbohydrates, like white sugar and white flour, wreak havoc with your blood sugar balance and rob you of real energy. They are "energy bandits." Consumption of regular quantities of refined sugar can lead to disglycemia and other blood sugar disturbances. Extreme disturbances can lead to type 2 diabetes.

THREE REASONS WHY SUGAR IS BAD FOR YOU

The first reason why sugar is bad for you is that too much sugar can be toxic and disrupt your blood sugar balance. Although glucose itself is not toxic, if your blood sugar level goes above the maximum threshold (as in disglycemia and diabetes), glucose becomes toxic to the brain. This is why diabetics develop nerve, eye, and brain damage.

Blood sugar disturbances create symptoms like fatigue, irritability, dizziness, insomnia, excessive sweating, poor concentration, forgetfulness, excessive thirst, depression, digestive disturbances, and blurred vision.

The second reason why sugar is bad for brain health is that it depletes your body's vital supply of vitamins and minerals and gives you back...well, nothing. Sugar is one of the most notorious energy bandits; it is an empty nutrient, it has zero value for your body, and it can create a breeding ground for bad cells like cancer and yeast infections like candida.

The third reason to avoid sugar excess is that high consumption is linked to poor mental health and lower IQ. This is why white sugar is not on the menu for a high-performance brain.

According to researchers at Massachusetts Institute of Technology, the higher the intake of refined carbohydrates, the lower your IQ. The research showed that the low-sugar consumers tested 35 points higher in IQ tests versus high-sugar consumers. Other studies revealed a worrisome link between high sugar consumption and behavioral problems like aggression, anxiety, hyperactivity, and attention deficit, as well as learning disabilities and fatigue.[42,43,44]

The following conditions are associated with high sugar consumption, proven conclusively by research at MIT and by Dr. Carl Pfeiffer, the founder of Princeton University's Brain Bio Center: aggressiveness, anxiety, hyperactivity, Attention Deficit Disorder, eating disorders, fatigue, learning disabilities, schizophrenia, as well as antisocial, fearful, phobic, psychotic and suicidal behavior.[45]

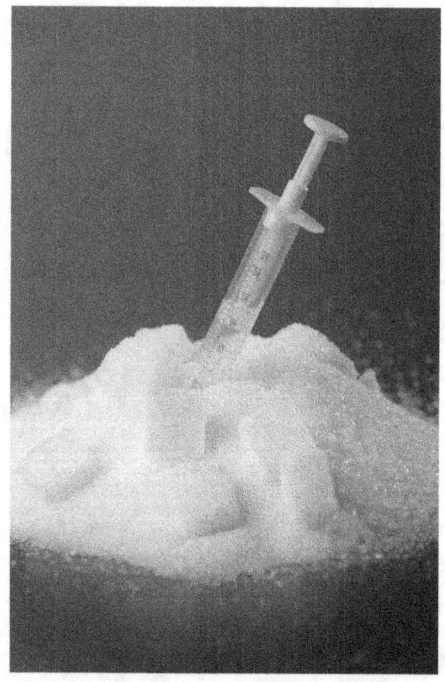

Sugar "Crack" Is the Twenty-First-Century Addiction

Sugar addiction has been on the rise since the last century as more foods contain higher levels of sugar. Conventional wisdom tells you to lower your fat intake. The lower fat intake reduces your ability to feel satiated, and the lack of real nutrients in your food keeps your body craving energy, so you turn to sugar, your favorite instant glucose hit, your energy "crack," when you feel tired, depressed, or sad.

There is a flip side to this coin, because blood sugar problems are related to stimulants and stress. When blood sugar levels go down, you look for ways to raise it. One way to do this is to eat foods that give you a glucose rush. The other way is to increase your adrenaline and cortisol (hormones produced in reaction to stress) by drinking tea or coffee, eating chocolate, or smoking cigarettes.

As Holford points out, this creates a vicious cycle of sugar, stress, and stimulants. You wake up each morning with low blood sugar levels, so you drink a caffeinated drink, usually coffee, to jumpstart your energy and get rid of the brain fog often caused by addiction to caffeine.

A refined carb (doughnut, toast, bagel, etc.) gives you a sugar rush, raising your blood sugar and adrenaline levels so you can function and feel normal. You go through the day with continuous dips of energy because you are not consuming enough complex carbohydrates, vitamins, and mineral nutrients to boost your energy enzymes. You are not eating quality fat to help you feel full, so you look to fast-burning carbs and lots of stimulants to get you through the day—then the cycle repeats: sugar, stress, and stimulants.

Studies also show that high sugar consumption correlates with increased use of alcohol and can lead to alcoholism.

This is not a picture of high-performance health. If you resemble this pattern in any way, it is time to reinvent the new, healthier, high-performance you.

BRAIN FUEL FOR HIGH PERFORMANCE

Any concentrated effort—spending ten hours a day in the office, making a presentation, driving a car, or solving a crossword puzzle—is directly affected by the food you eat throughout the day.

What foods should you eat to improve brain performance and health? Remember that there are two sides to the health coin. There are foods you should include in your diet to optimize brain health, and there are foods you need to avoid.

The food categories to include in your diet for optimal brain performance are as follows:

1) **Glucose**. As mentioned, brains are hogs. They consume 60 percent of the energy you have, and glucose is your brain fuel. To use the race car metaphor, you need high-quality fuel for your brain, not diesel, not regular gas, but high-octane, high-quality glucose from complex carbohydrates (whole grains, legumes, vegetables, and low-glycemic fruits).

2) **Essential fats.** The essential fats play a critical role in the brain's ability to process and send and receive information. Think of your brain as a high-speed computer that NASA uses to send rockets to the moon. You need the function of a RAM memory and processor to have speed and memory capacity. Essential fats are like processor chips; they give your brain speed and keep it well lubricated so that it can function efficiently (think fish, olive oil, and walnuts).

3) **Amino acids** from proteins (fish, lentils, tofu, beans, quinoa, poultry, beef, and eggs). The correct amino acids can help you feel motivated and happy, and they assist you when you need to navigate stressful circumstances (remember that the US military has research on this). Conversely, if you don't give your body the right raw materials, it cannot manufacture the

right hormones in the correct amounts to satisfy your brain requirements.

4) **Intelligent micronutrients** found in vitamins and minerals (fruits, vegetables, herbs, and spices). Think of this group of nutrients as the brain's fine-tuners. They are essential to the manufacturing that goes on behind the scenes. They help turn glucose into energy and amino acids into neurotransmitters, and they turn essential fats into more complex fats that boost brain function.

5) **Phospholipids.** Phospholipids found in eggs, organ meats, and lecithin are the insulation in the wiring, and they improve the brain's ability to send the messages over one hundred million synapses and connections.

6) **Water.** The brain needs **high-quality water.** Turn off the tap water if you do not have a filter on it. Better yet, buy a high-quality alkaline drinking water filtration system that can provide an alkalinizing effect on your body.

THE FLIP SIDE OF THE BRAIN-HEALTH COIN

Just as there are foods that improve brain performance, there are foods that harm the brain, its performance, and long-term health.

1. **Bad fats.** Excessive intake of saturated fats in red meats, dairy, packaged and fried foods.

2. **Refined sugar and refined carbohydrates:** all packaged foods, and most white foods.

3. **Alcohol:** This may come to some as a surprise, but alcohol is not a health food.

4. **Stimulants:** Caffeine, sugar, tobacco.

Knowing both sides of the superior health equation is essential if you are to succeed on the road to high performance.

Now that you know what categories of nutrients you need to sharpen your brain health and performance, and the categories that diminish your brain's competencies, the next step is to become the architect and engineer for your "house" of health. Learn about your construction materials—what foods give these nutrients—so you can prepare your shelves, and your mind, and seek them out.

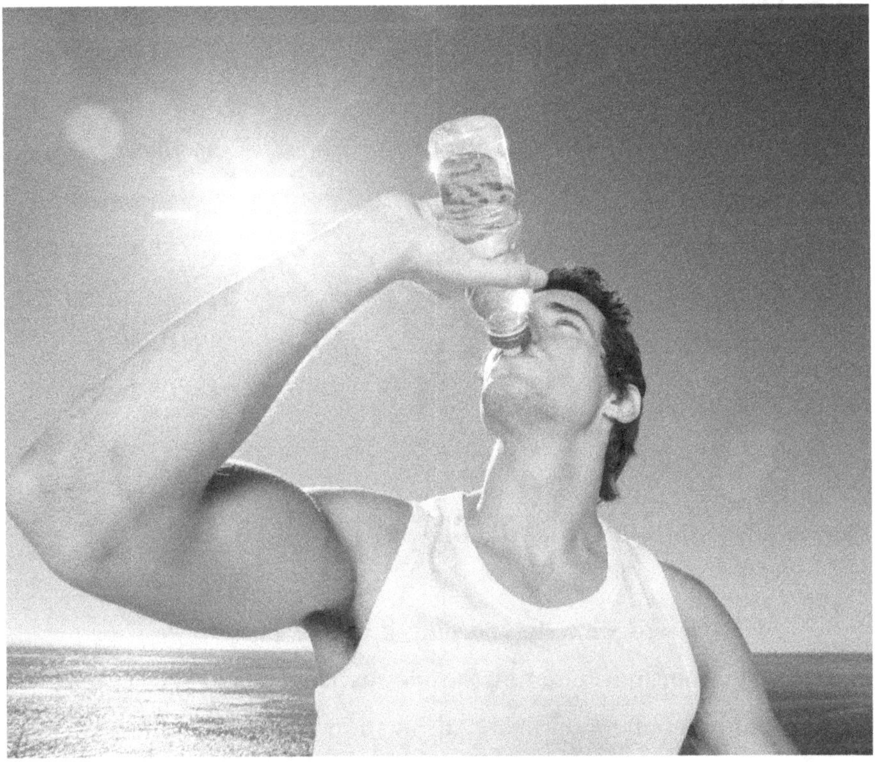

CHAPTER 5:

✡ ✡ ✡

THE BASICS OF CELLULAR ENERGY OPTIMIZATION (CEO) HEALTH

STEP 5: LEARN THE SEVEN BASICS FOR SUPERIOR HEALTH.

"Live in rooms full of light. Avoid heavy food. Be moderate in the drinking of wine. Take massage, baths, exercise, and gymnastics. Fight insomnia with gentle rocking or the sound of running water. Change surroundings and take long journeys. Strictly avoid frightening ideas. Indulge in cheerful conversation and amusements. Listen to music." —**A. Cornelius Celsus**

RECIPE FOR OPTIMAL HEALTH

We want to simplify and amplify how you achieve superior health by pointing out some basic information that allows you to create your program for optimal health within a workable framework.

The fundamental principle of superior health is optimizing the performance of the cells in your body, which create better functioning organs, systems, and better overall physiology. The basic requirements are the following high-quality ingredients:

1)   *Water*
2)   *Air*
3)   *Sleep*
4)   *Sun*
5)   *Recharging*
6)   *Fuel*
7)   *Exercise*

The key words in the prescription are high quality, because as you know, there are different grades of quality for each element. You may have noticed by now the point that we are hammering into your consciousness: To achieve high performance, emphasize the quality of basic fuels and the energy supply for your body and be vigilant about "energy bandits."

Two other dimensions of superior health include maintaining balance and removing waste and toxins (detoxification), the elements that disrupt balance.

The body and brain operate as a complex system of interactions that boggle the mind, but what keeps them in good shape is simple. Remember that the body and brain are made from molecules that come from food, air, sun, and water. It makes sense that your health, and the optimal functioning of your operating systems, depends on the quality supply of those four ingredients.

Add to this the critical time period when the "night crew" (sleep) cleans and repairs the internal cells, the need to assist circulation of lymph and other bodily fluids that maintain the health of the organs (exercise), the recuperative process of relaxation that supports immunity and psychological balance (recharging), and the essential sanitation work that involves identifying, neutralizing, and removing toxins and molecular waste products (detoxification), and you have the recipe for optimal health. How hard can this be? Yet somehow we fail to learn these basics, and/or we neglect to pay attention to them in our daily lives.

For example, we need to learn more about our basic water supply. If the water we are drinking is contaminated with antibiotics and treated with chemicals that endanger our health, the water is not high quality. Similarly, averaging four to five hours of sleep a night does not meet the standard of quality for high performance; we should strive for seven to eight hours of uninterrupted sleep each night.

This prescription for improving health may sound too simple or obvious, and therefore not plausible in a world where people are programmed to seek a pill for every ailment. Achieving health and sustaining it *is* simple if you don't allow yourself to get tangled up in poor habits, based on misconceptions that lead to deteriorating health.

So, let's untangle the misconceptions and set the record straight.

THE CELL: ENGINE FOR ENERGY

We begin with a look at the most basic component of life, the cell. If you optimize the energy of the cell, you get the whole health engine humming. It's what we call Cellular Energy Optimization (CEO).

Every organ in your body—skin, teeth, muscles, kidneys, heart, and bones—is made of cells. Cells make up your tissues and organs and the operating systems of your body.

Cells are like factories for energy production. They are programmed for specific use, depending on their DNA coding, but they all deliver energy to carry out their responsibilities. Cells that make up your kidney carry out purification and elimination; cells that make up your heart carry out the job of pumping and carrying the electrical signals necessary to keep it beating in a rhythmic way; cells that make up your liver are programmed to deliver energy for detoxifying and neutralizing poisons so that your organs are not harmed.

The cell is the basic unit of life. If the energy work in the cells is functioning at full capacity, the body is in better condition, because the organs and systems they make up (cardiovascular, respiratory, etc.) work at optimal efficiency. When an organ malfunctions, millions of cells are malfunctioning.

Cells depend upon many things for optimal function. Oxygen, for example, is necessary to manufacture energy. Amino acids from protein sources are used for repair or to replace worn-out cells. When a cell is deprived of the substances it needs to function, it dies, becomes acidic waste, and is eliminated, or it can adapt to the lack of oxygen and nutrients and become malignant.

Given that each cell is programmed to release energy, when it can no longer provide energy due to lack of oxygen, it uses fermentation, a process that releases energy without oxygen. As it multiplies, it harvests nutrients from healthier cells. The normal cells, which have been victims of nutrient theft from malfunctioning cells, stop dividing and die. This is the process of diseases like cancer.[46]

Dr. Roger Williams, a biochemist who conducted research on nutrients in food in the last century, asserted that the major cause of disease was not bacteria or viruses but cellular malnutrition. His assertions were backed up by research on yeast cells. The cells showed that the efficiency with which each cell carries out its metabolic duties was a direct function of nutritional status.[47] Williams also showed that cells die not only because of lack of nutrients but also because of toxins from chemical additives.

If your cells are healthy, your organs and operating systems are usually healthy. If the basic unit of life is not healthy because it is not getting what it needs (nutrition, water, oxygen), or its ability to do its job has been compromised by toxins, damage, or radiation, your health is compromised.

THE WONDERS OF WATER

Water is usually the nutrient that is in short supply in the body, leading to a wide range of health problems that may not seem obvious at first but show up as small signals (headaches, aches and pains, and peptic ulcers).[48]

People rarely invest time in thinking about what they drink, unless it's what wine they order with dinner, which soda with lunch, or the next coffee break.

The single most important nutrient in your diet is not the carbs that you love or the amount of vegetables you consume daily, but the quality and amount of water you drink.

Pure, clean water is *the* most essential nutrient in your life. This does not mean coffee, tea, soda, or anything with sugar or caffeine—this means unadulterated water. Water is so important to survival that fewer than five days without water can result in death, and an inadequate intake (a deficiency of less than 1 percent) can severely compromise health and result in dysfunction.

What substance do you know that can exist in three distinct forms (solid, liquid, or gas) and has a range of 100 degrees before it boils? Water is so whacky that as ice, it becomes less dense, whereas most substances become denser when frozen. This is good, because otherwise water wouldn't freeze and float at the surface of ponds and lakes. It would freeze under, killing all the life in it, because its heaviness would cause it to sink and expand upward. If water didn't have an extensive range as a liquid form, blood would literally boil on a hot summer's day.

So, the question that we need to ask is: Why is water so important?

It is helpful to our understanding of how the body works that we know this answer, and that we understand exactly what water does, so we can appreciate its multitudinous.

KING OF MULTITASKING

Water participates in all of the life-sustaining chemical reactions that enable you to function. It is the "king of multitasking" in your body. It has so many roles that when it comes to productivity, it is unsurpassed.

Every function of the body is monitored and pegged to the efficient flow of water. Any decrease in your daily water intake affects the efficiency of cell activity.[49]

A partial list of the more important roles water has in the health of the cells follows:

1) **Regulates metabolism.** Water has an essential hydrolytic role in all aspects of metabolism and all water–dependent chemical reactions. This means that water is responsible for all chemical reactions that create and sustain life. The "hydrolytic role" is the decomposition of any chemical compound by reaction with water, which is what happens every time you eat. If it were not for this function, you would not be able to break down the proteins in steak or chicken, for example, and absorb the nutrients of amino acids into your cells.

2) **Hydroelectric energy generator.** The flow of water through the cell membrane can generate hydroelectric energy, which is then stored in the energy pools of the cell "battery" systems. All cells have unique sources of energy known as adenosine triphosphate (ATP) and guanosine triphosphate (GTP). The energy in these "battery" systems is used for basic exchanges, particularly in neurotransmission. *When you feel tired and reach for a caffeinated drink, it could be that you are not giving your cells enough water to generate energy.*[50]

3) **Adhesive.** Water forms a structural pattern and shape that seems to be used as an adhesive material in bonding the cell architecture. It attaches the solid structures of the cell membrane, developing the stickiness of ice at higher body

temperatures. "This property of water makes it possible for life to regenerate itself on the DNA assembly line in a series of "protected" and walled environments-thoroughly protected environments within other environments."[51]

4) **Transportation.** Water is the primary mode of transportation in the body; your body is 60 percent water, and your blood is close to 90 percent. Without water, your body cannot move nutrients into the cells and waste products out of them. The less water you drink, the more waste accumulates in our blood and organs. David Wolfe, raw food enthusiast, said of the waste accumulation impact of not drinking water, "If you do not dilute, you pollute."

5) **Solvent.** Water can dissolve more substances than any other liquid. This property allows your body to assimilate nutrients and neutralize other substances.

6) **Body hydration.** To repeat, your body is 60 percent water, and every part of you consists of water: blood is close to 90 percent, the brain is 85 percent, and even bones are 30 percent. When you deplete internal water without replenishing it, you become dehydrated, which is extremely damaging to the joints, tendons, intestines, kidneys, heart, brain and other organs of the body.

7) **Extraction.** Water extracts nutrients from food so that they can be transported to the cells.

8) **Nourishment and replenishment of vital fluids.** All the fluids in your body, including lymph, intracellular fluid, and

the internal environment of each cell, consist of water. Water hydrates and lubricates the tissues and delivers nutrients into the cells.

9) **Cleansing and detoxification.** Water's ability to act as solvent and transporter allows it to work with the immune system to cleanse your internal environment and flush unwanted toxins.

10) **Lubrication.** Water keeps joints lubricated so that they work better. If you are experiencing problems with your knees and/or back (not injury related), then pay attention to how much water you consume during the day, every day.

11) **Keeps you "regular."** Water's role as solvent and transporter moves fiber and debris through the intestines until they are safely removed.

12) **Supports the liver.** Water helps the liver metabolize fat and purify toxins.

13) **Brain fuel.** If you want a high-performance brain, water is one of your most important allies. Because the brain is 85 percent water, you need water to optimize brain function and achieve high performance.

All bodily functions depend on water, including but not limited to the metabolism of fat, the lubrication of our joints, the production of energy, the transportation of nutrients into the cells, and all the activities mentioned.

Without sufficient water, you become dehydrated, which leads to fatigue, sugar cravings, and edginess. Because culture and food habits have led us more toward caffeinated and carbonated beverages with a high sugar content and/or adulterated sugar substitutes, all of which dehydrate the cells, most people are chronically dehydrated.

THE DANGERS OF DEHYDRATION

DO YOU WANT YOUR CELLS TO LOOK LIKE LUSCIOUS GRAPES OR LIKE RAISINS?

Take a look at your daily liquid intake. Most people don't realize that they are not drinking the minimum eight glasses of water a day (2,500–3,000 milliliters). More is required with exercise, illness, hot weather, and indoor living. If you drink other beverages like a Starbucks caramel latte, black tea, a diet Coke, or sweetened juice, you think, "There is water in these drinks, so doesn't this count toward my eight glasses?"

The answer is no. These drinks are dehydrating, and some of them are diuretics, meaning they cause you to lose fluids (like anything caffeinated), and this is not good for your body or your brain.[52]

To reiterate, the body is 60 percent water, and water is required for almost all bodily functions. When you become dehydrated, your cells, organs, systems, and most importantly, your brain do not work as well as they should. The cells start to lose water. Picture a bunch of luscious, plump grapes; that is the picture of your cells fully hydrated and in full operating condition. Now think of a handful of raisins. These are your cells when you deprive them of water, still edible but not functioning well. The net result is that you get symptoms with "raisin" cells. The symptoms are small at first, but over time, as your body craves water, the symptoms increase.

As soon as the body is deprived of water, it starts rationing water to protect the vital organs and keep everything working. Histamine, a neurotransmitter, becomes more active and redistributes water throughout the body (the order of priority is the brain, lungs, liver, kidneys, glands, muscles, bones, and skin).

During dehydration, histamine makes sure that the vital organs have enough water to keep working, but if water is not supplied, it must be taken from within the body. Chronic dehydration causes this neurotransmitter to become excessively active, and this leads to the symptoms that you might mistakenly attribute to other disorders.

These are some of the symptoms associated with low-level, chronic dehydration (symptoms affecting thinking and decision making appear in bold):

- Allergies
- Asthma
- **Brain fog**
- Colitis
- Constipation
- **Concentration problems**
- Rheumatoid arthritis
- Chronic pains in various parts of the body
- **Low energy**
- **Memory loss**
- Migraine headaches
- Dyspeptic pain: heartburn, gastroesophageal reflux disorder (GERD)
- **Depression**
- **Tiredness**

With chronic dehydration, the natural signal for thirst *disappears*, but it comes back if you address it by drinking the correct amount of water each day. This point is worth highlighting: your signal for thirst disappears after years of dehydration. This means that you may not even be aware that you need to drink more water because you do not feel thirsty. If you fall into this category, start to count how many glasses of pure water you drink to ensure you are getting the minimum amount of eight glasses a day.

Dyspeptic pain (indigestion and upset stomach) is one of the early signs of dehydration. Water is critical to the digestive process when food enters the stomach and hydrochloric acid is secreted to activate the enzymes, which break down the proteins in meat and dairy.

The acidic contents of the stomach (chyme) are pumped into the small intestine, and it passes through a valve called the pyloric sphincter. This acid, because it is strong, must be neutralized so that it doesn't damage the intestinal lining. The pancreas secretes bicarbonate ions that neutralize the acid, but you need a lot of water to produce this neutralizing bicarbonate solution.

Without sufficient water, the digestive process can be delayed. Food stays in the stomach longer than it should, and stomach acid can enter the esophagus, producing the sensation known as heartburn.

Another common complication of dehydration is joint pain. Because cartilage, including that in your joints, consists of mostly water, the cells in cartilage become worn down without proper lubrication. As the exposed cells, which are constantly sliding and gliding over one another, become irritated and worn, they peel away. New cartilage is normally produced to replace the damaged cells, but due to the lack of blood vessels in cartilage, it relies on water to transport the nutrients.

Dehydration interferes with the process. The result is an increase in abrasive damage, delay in repair, and joint pain.

Three other common disorders can be symptoms of chronic dehydration: constipation, asthma, and allergies.

Constipation is easy to figure out. We get clogged, and there isn't enough water in the water system to "move the trash out." When water is in short supply, the colon restricts unnecessary water loss through the stools. Colon muscles contract to squeeze out and subsequently reabsorb water back into circulation. This can result in harder stools that are not only more difficult to pass but may irritate and weaken the walls of the colon, resulting in small pockets known as diverticuli. Because the water that the colon reabsorbs into circulation is waste water, the liver and the kidneys must filter it, placing additional strain on these organs.

Allergies and asthma are outcomes of chronic dehydration and an indication that the body is producing too much histamine. Because the body is trying to prevent unnecessary water loss, it constricts bronchial muscles to restrict water loss through expiration. This is because you lose a large amount of water through the lungs as water vapor.

Think about those raisins again. They are the reason to drink plenty of clean, pure water. Besides drinking eight glasses of pure water a day, drink a glass of water twenty minutes before every meal.

BEAUTY ON THE OUTSIDE FROM THE GRAPES ON THE INSIDE

Dehydration causes your cells to shrivel on the inside, so what do you think happens to the skin on the outside? Wrinkles. The lack of water inside and outside your cell walls shrinks the tissues; your skin cannot stay supple because there is not enough moisture in your cellular structure. You can dump as much moisturizer as you want on it, but it is not going to change your skin's destiny. Without water, your skin will dehydrate. If your cells shrivel like raisins, your face will too.

Water isn't the only ingredient in supple skin, but it is a major factor. Other major factors which contribute to wrinkles are smoking and sugar.

GARBAGE FLOATING INSIDE YOUR EXTRACELLULAR FLUIDS

The second reason for avoiding dehydration is "garbage" removal. Most of the body's water is found within the cells, and the next-largest amount is in the fluid surrounding the cells. If you are not replacing your cell water frequently, the surrounding fluid will continue to accumulate waste material and toxins. The pumps in the cell membranes cannot work efficiently because you are clogging the cell with dirty water, which can lead to cell damage or death. You wouldn't think of using bath water over and over without changing it, but that is exactly what is happening in your body when you do not drink enough clean water.[53]

Drink at least two to three quarts of water daily to achieve maximum brain function and high-performance physiology, and if you drink coffee or tea with caffeine, add two glasses for every cup. Don't forget that water needs to circulate, which requires you to move (hence, the importance of exercise).

AIR IS A NUTRIENT, AND BREATHING IS ITS VEHICLE

You can go forty-five days without food, and three to five days without water, but unless you have trained to hold your breath like an Olympic diver, a few minutes without air will result in your demise. In the scheme of life's essentials, air is at the top of the list. Getting air is not the question, because we all breathe without questioning the air supply. The real question to ask is, why is it so important to get the correct quantity of air into your body?

THE OXYGEN FACTOR

Like food and water, which are broken into components and used to produce energy and perform functions, air consists of oxygen, which drives the chemical reactions essential for sustaining and performing functions.

Red blood cells, circulation of nutrients, and numerous other functions of the body depend on oxygen:

1) Oxygen is essential for the proper functioning of the immune system; a shortage of oxygen therefore results in a breakdown of your immune system.

2) All nutrients—proteins, carbohydrates, fats, vitamins, and minerals—are used to create energy, and oxygen must be present.

3) Cells use oxygen to break down toxic substances.

4) Without oxygen, you cannot metabolize substances; therefore there is no nourishment and no energy for your cells. Oxygen is vital to the breakdown of glucose in each cell

In short, every bodily process uses oxygen.

The next critical question, therefore, is not whether you are breathing but if you are taking in sufficient air to allow you to nourish your cells. Are you obtaining an adequate level of oxygen to optimize your health?

The answer to this question is usually no. Most people have lost their innate ability to breathe properly, that is to say, from their diaphragm. Diaphragmatic breathing occurs when you breathe into the lower portion of your belly. If you are doing it right, your belly protrudes when you inhale.

Unless you pull the correct amount of oxygen into your body, your cells cannot obtain the necessary nutrients they need to create energy.

BREATHING IS THE BRIDGE BETWEEN BODY AND MIND

Breathing is not only the bridge between the body and the mind, it is the only vital autonomic function that you can control consciously. You never think about breathing, certainly not as much as you think about what you eat or what you do or don't do.

Breathing is not just the vehicle for transporting oxygen. It has numerous other functions that enhance health:

1) It harmonizes the functional systems of the body by pumping fresh supplies of blood and energy to vital organs.

2) It enhances mental clarity.

3) *It improves cerebral function.*

If you doubt this, try this exercise. Next time you are upset, angry, or stressed, notice how you are breathing. The breath grows short and shallow. It stays in the upper chest, and your diaphragm and abdomen do not move.

Most adults, particularly adults who live in cities, tend to breathe high in their chests, using the upper ribs and clavicle to suck in air into the smaller spaces at the top of the lungs.

Clavicular (upper chest) breathing is extremely inefficient and usually is an emergency response to stressful circumstances. It is the type of breathing associated with the "fight or flight" instinct.

For most adults, clavicular breathing is habitual. It seriously compromises your ability to circulate adequate oxygen into your blood, thereby straining your heart.

Your heart pumps two thousand gallons a day, one to six gallons per minute. In your lifetime, your heart pumps a million barrels! Without the necessary oxygen that breathing provides, the heart is strained by the load.[54]

Observe a baby when it sleeps. Its belly moves; the abdomen expands in inhalation and distends with exhalation while the chest remains still. Now observe your own chest when you breathe. Watch your chest move with each inhalation. Better still, the next time when you are with a group of people, particularly in a meeting in an office, watch to see if people breathe with their chest or diaphragm. Most people who work in white collar offices breathe with their chest.

Dr. A. Salmanoff described the diaphragm as the most powerful muscle in the body. By using your diaphragm, you take the pressure off the heart, which has to work against gravity.[55] His explanation is simple. The pressure from the diaphragm, when it is engaged properly during breathing, acts like a pump to drive stale blood from your internal organs through one of the major arteries (the vena cava) to the chest. This action saves the heart from expending enormous amounts of energy. The diaphragm becomes, in effect, a "second heart" that helps drive circulation.

Deep, abdominal breathing takes on the work of pumping blood to the brain, thereby enhancing circulation and acting as an accelerant for thinking.

Deep breathing has other benefits that support health:

1)   **Less stress and anxiety**. "Fight or flight" breathing is your fall back when you feel anxiety, making it automatic. Once

you switch to deep, abdominal breathing, consciously taking slow, deep breaths, the nervous system switches the action circuits from "fight or flight" mode to the parasympathetic system, the "rest and relax" mode.

2) **Increased lung capacity.** For every extra millimeter of flexing you do on inhalation with deep breathing, the diaphragm develops more range, increasing your lung capacity by 250–300 milliliters. According to studies in China, after six months of breathing practice, the diaphragm can increase its average flex by 4 millimeters, which results in an expanded lung capacity of 1,000-2,000 milliliters.[56] When you expand your lung capacity, you have better circulation, and the cells of our body become more efficient.

3) **Red blood cell activity increases.** After thirty minutes of regulated, deep breathing, the flow of oxygen to the cells improves.

4) **Digestion improves.** One session of deep breathing improves the digestive functions. Deep breathing stimulates secretions of bile, pepsin, and other digestive juices in the liver, stomach, and pancreas, and it improves the contractions that move waste products through the large intestine.

5) **Natural detox.** Deep breathing activates the body's innate cleansing and healing responses and triggers the release of neurotransmitters and hormones that tell the body to detoxify.

6) **Calms the nervous system and reduces blood pressure.** Deep breathing signals the nervous system to repair and

detoxify. By switching from the sympathetic to the parasympathetic branch of the nervous system, it has the effect of lowering blood pressure.

Although all the benefits of deep breathing are important, the last benefit, calming the nervous system and reducing blood pressure, is something you can control when you want to stay centered. We encourage you to put this tool into your HP toolbox.

SLEEP: REPAIR, RENEW, AND REWIRE YOUR BRAIN

"NO SLEEP MEANS NO NEW BRAIN CELLS"

An equally important and often undervalued tool for calming your central nervous system is sleep—the time the body uses to process the day and renew energy potential.

According to experts, sleep is critical for maintaining optimal health. Without it, you become more susceptible to heart disease, stroke, diabetes, obesity, and depression.

Recent studies showed that not getting adequate hours of uninterrupted sleep each night produced deficits in new brain cell production because of higher levels of the stress hormone corticosterone.

Studies showed that even small decreases in sleep, a little less every night, had the same effect and results in higher levels of this stress hormone, and lower levels of brain cell production.

According to sleep expert Dr. Neil Stanley, when an animal's corticosterone levels were kept at a constant level, "the reduction in cell proliferation was abolished, suggesting that the elevation in stress hormone levels resulting from sleep deprivation reduces cell production in the adult brain."[57]

Eventually, if sleep patterns are restored to normal, levels of nerve cell production (neurogenesis) are restored.

Another study, conducted by a team from Princeton University, found that a lack of sleep affected the hippocampus, the region involved in forming memories.

Still another research study, led by Dr. Elizabeth Gould, revealed that although the role of nerve cell production in adults remained unknown, "the suppression of adult neurogenesis may underlie some of the cognitive deficits associated with prolonged sleep deprivation."[58]

"Cognitive deficits:" a term we should all be concerned about. It refers to the diminishment of abilities. Specifically, it refers to all the problems you develop with mental acuity as your brain ages: diminished memory, concentration, and attention. Whether you are striving for a high-performance brain or just a normal life, avoid doing anything that results in those dreaded *cognitive deficits*.

LACK OF SLEEP AND HEALTH PROBLEMS

According to the September 2006 issue of *Archives of Internal Medicine*,[59] a lack of shut-eye makes people more susceptible to health problems.

Dr. Phyllis Zee and Fred Turek of Northwestern University Feinbery School of Medicine in Chicago reported that sleeplessness may harm the immune system.[60] According to their research, lack of sleep was linked to an increase in a molecule called a cytokine that controls immune responses. The increase in cytokines caused an inflammatory response and changes in blood chemistry, which were linked to heart disease, diabetes, and neurological conditions.

According to a report published by the Institute of Medicine, which is comprised of the nation's leading scientists on health issues, sleep problems and the cumulative effects of sleep deprivation "represent an under recognized public health problem" and are associated with a wide range of health issues, including increased risk of obesity, Type 2 diabetes, high blood pressure, depression, stroke, and heart attack.[61]

Another study of fourteen hundred middle-aged adults found that those with sleep apnea (a condition whereby the airway becomes repeatedly blocked and sleep is interrupted) were twice as likely to develop depression.

Dr. Damien Léger of Assistance Publique Hôpitaux de Paris found a higher rate of sleep problems and daytime sleepiness among allergy sufferers, compared with a control group of people of the same age and sex who lived in the same area. According to Léger, "The results show a significant impact of allergic rhinitis on all dimensions of sleep quality and, consequently, a lower quality of life as reflected by more somnolence [sleepiness], daytime fatigue and sleepiness, and impaired memory, mood and sexuality."[62]

As reported in *Archives of Internal Medicine*, other studies concluded that men with diabetes and men with short- or poor-quality sleep tended to have less control of their blood-sugar levels. "The foundations of good health are good diet, good exercise and good sleep, but two out of three doesn't get you there," said Dr. Anne Calhoun, a neurology professor at the University of North Carolina.

NIGHT CREW DOES REPAIR WORK DURING SLEEP

Think of your body as a manufacturing facility. The cells in each organ are programmed for specific tasks that facilitate a specific function. For example, your respiratory organs are involved in taking in oxygen and expelling carbon dioxide, which is moved by your circulatory system (blood, arteries, vessels), which gains momentum from the cardiovascular system (heart-pumping action with a network of veins and capillaries).

Throughout the day, the crews work to provide you the energy to think, move, digest, work, and play. After the work is done for the day, it's time for the clean-up, maintenance, and repair night crew to rebuild or replace cells that are worn out, remove waste, and get things ready for another day.

The night crew can do its job only when the systems shut down for the night—when you sleep. If your mind and body are still expending energy when they should be sleeping, the body does not have time to do the maintenance work, and this is critical to your ability to maintain good health.

One of the main processes that takes place at night, specifically when your systems shut down to start repair, is troubleshooting for toxins that look like innocent molecules but are really dangerous and uninvited participants. This is called detoxification, and it is one of the body's most important functions.

Here are a few facts about the importance of a good night's sleep. (Adapted from *Detoxification and Healing* by Dr. Sidney MacDonald Baker)

1) Everything in the body—all the molecules left over from the daily operations of the brain, bowels, blood, bones, muscles, skin, and internal organs—must be neutralized and/or rendered harmless and eliminated by detoxification.

2) Detoxification is the most costly metabolic activity of the body. Making the molecules for detoxification requires the lion's share of the energy you expend on making any kind of molecule every day.

3) If your machinery for detoxification (the liver) emitted noise while detoxifying, the grinding, groaning noise would be so loud

that it would drown out all other noises of everyday life. The molecular details of managing the identification and removal of toxins, allergens, and other wastes are pervasive in your body.

4) If your body were a municipality, and the detoxification function were your sanitation department, the budget for the department, in terms of energy expenditure (for cleansing, clean-up, maintenance and repair) would be 80 percent of the municipal budget![63]

This puts everything in perspective. Detoxification is an essential part of maintaining your health, and the bulk of it occurs while you sleep.

If you need to adjust your life to get more sleep, start now. Wrap up the paperwork, turn off the TV, finish the day's business well before you lie down for sleep, and allow your body time to get into sleep mode.

If you have a sleep disorder and have difficulty getting more than four or five hours of sleep a night, get it treated. Identify the possible causes, and find out what remedies are available. For example, if you drink several cups of caffeinated drinks during the day, try cutting back. Better yet, try eliminating caffeine and see if you see an improvement in your sleep patterns. If you are experiencing chronic stress, integrate some new stress management techniques into your daily schedule. Try multiple intervention strategies until you wrestle the problem to the ground and experience more satisfying sleep.

Sleep is one of the big items in your tool box for high performance. Pay attention to it.

SUNLIGHT IGNITES VITAMIN D AND HORMONE PRODUCTION

The main mechanism whereby sunlight provides nutrition is through skin exposure. Sunlight stimulates the tissues below the skin to produce vitamin D, which is an essential co-factor for assimilating and using calcium. Without vitamin D, the body cannot absorb calcium, and without calcium, the body cannot detoxify and repair itself.

It is one of the tragic consequences of modern lifestyles and urban living (in the West and the industrialized world) that people no longer get adequate exposure to clean, full-spectrum sunlight.

The proper daily "dosage" of sunlight is thirty minutes, taken before 10:30 a.m. or after 3:30 pm. In *Alkalize or Die,* Dr. Theodore Baroody states that you need one-half hour of direct sunlight a day for the body to produce the correct amounts of hormones and maintain correct alkaline acid balances.[64]

Artificial lighting, both fluorescent and incandescent, does not contain the full spectrum wavelength that exists in sunlight.

For most of human existence, the body had adequate access to full-spectrum light throughout the day. Today, many people work in office buildings, spend endless hours at desks or with their computer and iPhone, and they forget to go outside to get fresh air and sunlight.

Worse than this is the phobia about sun: people have been so sensitized to "the dangers" of sun (skin cancer) that sun is avoided or taken with large doses of sunblock and sunscreen. Sunscreens not only block sun exposure, but they are chemical cocktails with petroleum-based derivative substances that contribute to cellular degeneration and disease. The result is solar deficiency that contributes to calcium deficiency (the main reason that we see weak teeth and bones in adults today). This deficiency, also called mal-illumination, has many negative effects on health and well-being.

You need full-spectrum light because it is essential for the regulation of hormones (vitamin D has been reclassified as a hormone). It catalyses secretions from the pituitary gland, and the specialized hormones are responsible for regulating many body functions. Without full-spectrum light, you are deprived of the necessary stimulation of hormones, and your body cannot work at optimal efficiency.

Lack of full-spectrum light can wreak havoc with the absorption of dietary nutrients and lead to cellular degeneration and disease.

This last fact is worth repeating: lack of sufficient vitamin D results in cellular degeneration and disease. This has been proven. Without adequate sun, your body cannot manufacture essential vitamins, trigger the pituitary to secrete hormones, assist with the absorption of nutrients, and function at its highest level of health. Without sun and vitamin D, your health will deteriorate. (More details below)

VITAMIN D DEFICIENCY AND DISEASE

Dr. Joseph Mercola, author of *Dark Deception* and one of the leading proponents of vitamin D therapy, discusses the "epigenetic influences" of vitamin D in regulating two thousand out of the thirty thousand genes that have been identified in the body. Without this vitamin, only 10–15 percent of calcium ingested can be absorbed. With vitamin D, 80 percent of calcium is absorbed into the cells.[65]

Mercola's research indicates that vitamin D deficiencies are linked to autoimmune diseases such as rheumatoid arthritis, multiple sclerosis, and type 1 diabetes.

The benefits of adequate vitamin D levels are listed below:

- Acts as a potent antibiotic
- Increases antimicrobial peptides
- Decreases age-related DNA damage (with high levels)
- Lowers inflammatory responses

- Helps with psoriasis, eczema, insomnia, hearing loss, periodontal disease, myopia, pre-eclampsia, seizures, and fertility
- Increases brain health and brain performance
- **Stimulates neurotransmitters serotonin that make you feel happy (decreases depression)**

Perhaps the most outstanding benefit of vitamin D is its proven ability to reduce the incidence of cancer by inhibiting differentiation, invasiveness, proliferation, metastatic potential, and angiogenesis, the process by which new blood vessels form from pre-existing vessels. Vitamin D exposure from the sun reduces cancers of the breast, colon, prostate, lung (early stages); non-Hodgkin's lymphoma; and melanoma.

The antithesis is also revealed in research. Vitamin D deficiencies increase the risk of contracting these cancers, and even without symptoms, too little vitamin D is associated with increased risk of death from cardiovascular disease and cognitive impairment in older adults.[66]

Dr. Mercola supports his findings with research, which he shares on his website and in many interviews and lectures, so we encourage you to investigate this subject further. Vitamin D from sunlight is one of the least celebrated but one of the most important tools you have for optimizing health and achieving high performance. (http://www.mercola.com/).

If you are concerned that the sun will cause skin cancer, weigh the risk of contracting diseases associated with insufficient vitamin D against the danger of skin cancer. Fully investigate the chemicals in your sunblock, and determine which ones are petrochemical derivatives. Ask yourself if the rise in skin cancer as a result of sun exposure can be attributed to other toxins that disrupt the balance of health in your body. The dangers of absorbing petrochemicals through the skin (from suntan lotion) also pose significant risks to your health.

Be cautious, not phobic, about getting sun. Avoid getting sun between 10:30 a.m. and 3:30 p.m., wear a hat to protect the collagen in your face, and use only sunblocks with natural ingredients.

Sun makes you feel good, so enjoy as much as you can.

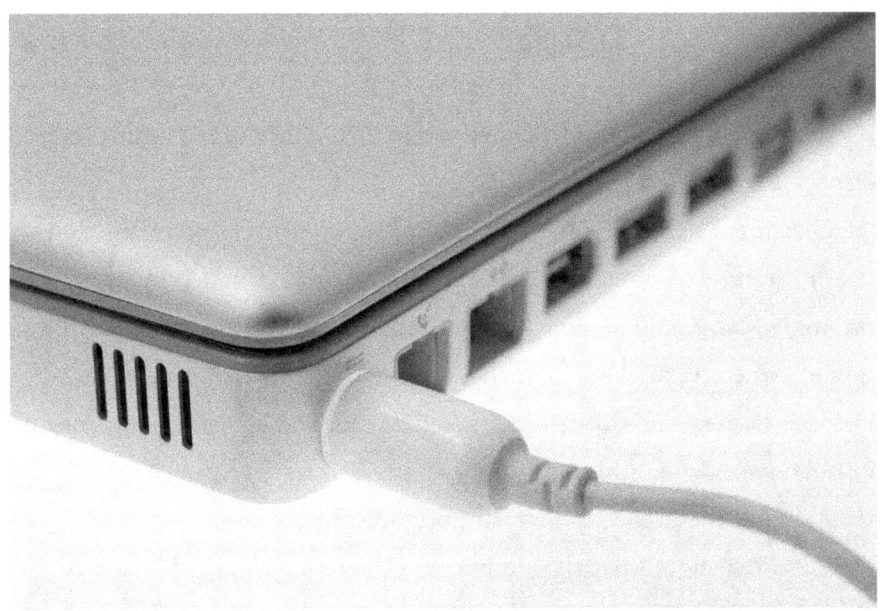

RECHARGE, OR YOUR BATTERIES WON'T WORK

We all have cellphones, smartphones, BlackBerrys, computers, iPads, and laptops and the necessary equipment to keep the batteries charged. If you don't recharge the batteries, the equipment doesn't work.

Your body is like a cellphone. If you forget to recharge, the battery depletes, and your health suffers.

Your cell phone might alert you of a low battery, and show you a picture of a battery cell. It's time to plug into an outlet for recharging. Unfortunately, you do not have an alert for your own "battery." When your batteries are depleted, you get signals, like headaches, and tiredness.

Stress rises. Your mood deteriorates. You are having less fun at whatever you are doing. Sometimes you get backup battery support from the adrenal glands, because you have learned to overstimulate them with caffeinated drinks and sugar, but in the end, your batteries stay depleted, and your performance and mood suffer.

Let's pretend for a minute that you have a battery signal. The battery signal would kick in at the end of each day and flash a warning: time to recharge. That would be the signal for six to eight hours of uninterrupted sleep.

Getting a good night's sleep when you are pushing your limits every day, running a company, running a family, or just managing your life, often gives you only a partial charge. Your mind and body keep running down at the end of the day until you take the time to stop and recharge and the battery cells read "100 percent." Instead of "plugging into an outlet," we advise "plugging out"—that is, completely separating from your environment psychologically and physically.

Research shows that the simple act of becoming relaxed can have surprising health benefits. Not only is there the well-recognized effect of relieving anxiety and mental tension, but there is also research to support that deep relaxation, especially if practiced regularly, can strengthen the immune system and produce a wide range of other valuable physiological changes.

For people with asthma, relaxation training has the impact of widening restricted respiratory passages. With some diabetics, relaxation can sometimes reduce the need for insulin. With chronic pain, many patients reveal that relaxation training helps relieve the symptoms, even when the pain is thought to be unbearable. Research also shows that relaxation helps ward off disease by making people less susceptible to viruses and by lowering blood pressure and cholesterol.[67]

Dr. Herbert Benson, the father of modern mind-body medicine, pioneered breakthrough research at Harvard Medical School. His research demonstrated that relaxation, which can be elicited through a variety of methods including but not limited to meditation, is the physiological counterpoint to the fight-or-flight response and is a natural antidote to stress.

In an interview with Daniel Redwood for the publication *Health Insights Today,* Benson described his research and the effect his technique, called the "relaxation response," has on physiological markers.[68] Specifically, he demonstrated that a series of physiologic indicators, which are increased by stress, can be decreased by practicing relaxation. These indicators included lowering metabolic and heart rate and reducing blood pressure, all of which are increased by stress.

He pointed out that 60–90 percent of doctor visits are related to stress and therefore respond poorly to treatment by drugs or surgery. The importance of this, he said, is that, "Our minds have the capability to bring forth a response opposite to the fight-or-flight response that could have therapeutic value."[69]

What is the magical relaxation response identified by his research?

It is not one single activity, like meditation, but a thread that weaves together repetitive behaviors so they become a means to an end, relaxing the mental landscape to the point where it can escape from negative thoughts. People have been doing these relaxation techniques for thousands of years, but we have lost a sense of their importance in the last five or six decades.

These techniques include yoga, meditation, repetitive prayer, tai chi, qigong, jogging, knitting, crocheting, building toy airplanes, sailing, gardening, painting—anything that effectively preoccupies the mind. All these activities have the effect of releasing the mind so that it can relax and calm the key physiological markers associated with stress.

What can you do to achieve this state of relaxation and enjoy the benefits of decreased metabolism and blood pressure, lowered heart rate, slower breathing, and slower brain waves?

Find the time. Overachievers and high performers are often overscheduled in their quest for super-productivity. To benefit from the simple strategy of relaxation, acknowledge its importance as a priority. Follow your passions and develop your hobbies. Make room in your daily program for activities that allow you to disengage from busy, mind-bending, anxiety- and/or stress-provoking, overstimulating routines. Make appointments at least five times a week with yourself (think of it as making time for a critical appointment with the doctor). Relaxation is an important part of your antistress arsenal, so spend at least thirty minutes a day with your passion or hobby, whether it is jogging, meditating, gardening, knitting, or praying.

The key finding in Benson's research is that relaxation must be repetitive (like a word, a sound, a prayer, a phrase, or a movement), and it must be consciously cultivated in order to free your thoughts from automatic negative thoughts (ANTs). Dr. Daniel Amen, quoted frequently because of his excellent research and author of *Use Your Brain to Change Your Age,* coined the term. ANTs can hold your mind hostage to negative and profoundly stressful mental patterns. To disperse ANTs, interrupt and redirect the train of thoughts that create stress and anxiety.

In Benson's interview, he described the relaxation technique as "breaking the train of everyday thought…it would appear that a fundamental entry point is the nervous system…the breaking of the train of everyday thought needn't be a mental effect; it could be a physical effect brought about by, say, jogging, knitting or crocheting. Are you with me? Ultimately, it's mediated through and by the nervous system."

Benson found that relaxation was effective with treatment of anxiety, mild and moderate depression, and excessive anger.

Be conscious of what you can do to break the train of your ANTs. Enjoy or develop a hobby, whether it's repairing clocks or automobiles, doing word games and puzzles, or learning tai kwon do. Do something that fits the criteria outlined here, and do it as often as you can or at least as often as necessary to keep your stress under control. This will help you balance your psychological and physical states, one of the keys to HP.

CHAPTER 6:

✡ ✡ ✡

CEO BASICS CONTINUED

STEP 5: LEARN THE BASICS: FUEL

"To eat is a necessity, but to eat intelligently is an art." —***La Rochefoucauld***

"Those who think they have no time for healthy eating, will sooner or later have to find time for illness." —***Edward Stanley***

"Today, more than 95% of all chronic disease is caused by food choice, toxic food ingredients, nutritional deficiencies and lack of physical exercise." —***Mike Adams***

FUEL FOR YOUR ENGINE: MICRONUTRIENTS, MACRONUTRIENTS, FUNCTIONAL FOODS, AND WATER

Fuel is central to how your brain works. The quality of fuel you have for the brain, which doubles as construction material for the wiring, insulation and cell tower communication (synapses), affects how you think, feel, and process information from your senses.

The same principle applies to your body: the higher the fuel quality, the higher the quality of your health and performance.

These are the three categories of fuel consumption:

1) Micronutrients, the molecules that your body needs for fine-tuning or turning cells on and off, like vitamins and minerals

2) Macronutrients, the molecules that your body uses for energy, manufacturing new and/or repairing old cells, as well as for making enzymes and immune fighters; these are carbohydrates, fats, and proteins

3) Water; we have already discussed its role in our bodies, but now we need to identify high-quality, functional water versus low-quality, contaminated water.

Each category contributes to how well your body works or doesn't. Getting two out of three won't work, so it's critical to identify which category is the weakest in your fuel portfolio and strengthen its role in your daily life.

Let's start with micronutrients, the undervalued superstars of nutrition, and usually the weakest link in our fuel repertoire. Since we already talked about their value with regard to the brain, a quick snapshot of their work here will just refresh your memory on their importance.

THE MAGIC OF MICRONUTRIENTS: VITAMINS, MINERALS AND PHYTONUTRIENTS

Micronutrients are behind the scenes, supporting the key macronutrient players. They are the vitamins and minerals that help turn glucose into energy, amino acids into neurotransmitters, and simple essential fats into complex omega-3 and omega-6 fats. EPA and GLA (eicosapentaenoic acid and gamma-linolenic acid) are dietary fats that help form the brain and nervous system, maintain the fluidity of blood, and create the structure of cell membranes.[70]

They are also responsible for the production of fats necessary for mental and emotional health, called prostaglandins. These are extremely active hormone-like substances.[71]

Micronutrients also consist of another category of chemicals found in plants, called phytonutrients. When your diet lacks these extremely versatile micronutrients, your health suffers because you run into trouble making the materials your body needs to function properly.

Let's look at prostaglandins as an example. The production of these hormone regulators depends on micronutrients like zinc, magnesium, biotin, and vitamin B6. This is the first step in the process. The second step requires selenium, vitamin C and niacin.[72] Scientists are just beginning to scratch the surface of what prostaglandins do in the body, but we know that you cannot manufacture them without the help of the behind-the-scenes micronutrients.

Just to give you a quick glimpse of their power and importance, here is the short list of what prostaglandins do in the body: they help relax blood vessels, lower blood pressure, maintain water balance, boost immunity, decrease inflammation and pain, and regulate blood sugar balance. Prostaglandins are powerful regulators; make sure that you have an ample supply of micronutrients to turn this hormone switch on.

MICRONUTRIENT STARVATION

Although micronutrients are critical for high-performing health, there is evidence to support the theory that highly processed diets are so devoid of vital micronutrients that Westernized populations are suffering from "micronutrient starvation." This may not be as obvious as vitamin deficiency diseases such as scurvy (a deficiency in vitamin C) or beriberi (a deficiency in thiamine or vitamin B), but leading health experts believe that micronutrient starvation is one of the leading causes for the demise in health in Westernized countries. The lack of sufficient micronutrients has had a devastating impact on health.

The category of micronutrients that most of us are familiar with, vitamins and minerals, are well known: B-complex vitamins, vitamin C, and minerals like calcium and zinc. Others are less familiar, like carotenoids and bioflavonoids. These naturally occurring plant compounds are a subset of a micronutrient category called phytonutrients. Because this group of micronutrients does not have an RDA, even though they are critical for high-performance health, it's not likely you will find them listed on the side of a cereal box.

Even if they are not listed in ingredient labels, seek foods that contain a high percentage of them, because they are critical players in your high-performance fuel tank.

THE BODY'S FINE-TUNERS, PHYTONUTRIENTS (OR PHYTOCHEMICALS): THINK COLOR

Phytonutrients, also called phytochemicals, are naturally occurring compounds found in fruits and vegetables. They are what create the bright colors.

These micronutrients are no accident of Mother Nature; they are nature's stealth weapon against harmful microbes, animals, insects, and ultraviolet radiation. For example, the potent sulphur compounds in garlic and onions act as bug repellents. Other compounds protect plants from bacteria, viruses, and other natural enemies. It stands to reason that when you eat foods containing these plant-protecting compounds, they protect you too—not from the bugs in your garden but from the oxidants (molecules that can produce free radicals), toxins, and free radicals (unstable atom(s) that can damage cells and are believed to accelerate the progression of cancer, cardiovascular disease and age related diseases). that wreak havoc with your cholesterol levels, the flexibility of your arteries, and your cells.

The discovery of phytonutrients has changed everything we know about food. We have identified more than nine hundred kinds, and it is estimated that hundreds more are still undiscovered. One serving of vegetables is believed to contain over one hundred different phytochemicals!

WHY SHOULD YOU CARE HOW MANY PHYTONUTRIENTS YOU EAT?

Let's count how many ways these amazing compounds help you achieve superior health:

- They help reduce cellular damage.
- They help prevent cancer cell replication.
- They help decrease cholesterol levels.
- They strengthen the immune system.
- They reduce inflammation.
- They help maintain healthy blood sugar levels.

Here is the kicker for HP health: they help keep your brain functioning optimally. Many scientists say that phytonutrients may have an even more important role than vitamins in promoting health and preventing disease.

Oats, a great complex carb, have long been known to lower cholesterol because of the dietary fiber they contain, but that is not the end of the story. Scientists now know that the natural phytonutrients they contain, which are 50 percent more powerful than vitamin E, reduce the risk of heart disease.

Abundant research suggests that these micronutrients not only give you powerful protection against molecular invaders, they also keep your health engine humming.

COLOR YOUR PLATE

Red: Tomatoes, red bell peppers, strawberries, and watermelon. These have lycopene, phytoene, phytofluene, and vitamin E. Clinical studies suggest that the anti-oxidant properties of lycopene have cancer-fighting properties. Beets and raspberries have anthocyanins, which research shows can lower blood pressure and improve circulation.

Green: Broccoli, spinach, leafy greens, and honeydew melon. These have lutein, which may help with vision and reduce the risk of macular degeneration, cataracts, and colon cancer. Cabbage, sauerkraut, kale, and chard have glucosinolates. Research suggests that this micro-helper reduces the risk of cancers of the breast, prostate, and stomach.

Orange/Yellow: Apricots, carrots, mangos, squash. These all have beta-carotene, which helps reduce risk of heart disease and cancer and protects against infection. Citrus fruits, such as lemons, oranges, grapefruits, and tangerines, have bioflavonoids that reduce the risk of cancer and heart disease while promoting healthy skin, teeth, and bones.

Purple: Blackberries and blueberries. These help the immune system fight cancer and heart disease, and studies suggest they can reduce the effects of age-related memory loss. Eggplants, plums, prunes and raisins have phenolics, which also slow aging.

ONE MORE WORD ABOUT PHYTONUTRIENTS

Phytonutrients are a subset of "functional foods." Functional food began as a concept in the 1980s in Japan, where their official definition is "foods for specified health use." They perform a function targeted to health enhancement.

Functional foods are the micronutrients and macronutrients that your body needs for biochemical reactions and maintenance and repair work. They contain cancer-fighting, immune-building compounds and ingredients that cut your risk for disease and chronic illnesses.

SPICE UP YOUR LIFE

Spices are a subset of functional foods. Unlike herbs, which come from the leaves of plants, spices are made from the buds, bark, fruits, roots, or seeds of plants, and they have amazing healing potential.

They contain an abundance of super phytochemicals, as well as free-radical scavengers, antioxidants. Turmeric, for example, is rich in a compound called curcumin. In animal studies, curcumin has been shown to reduce the risk of colon cancer by 58 percent. Other spices help neutralize harmful substances in the body, destroying their cancer-causing potential. Nutmeg, ginger, cumin, black pepper, and coriander have been shown to help block the effects of aflatoxin, a mold that can cause liver cancer.[73]

WHAT DID THE ANCIENTS KNOW THAT YOU DON'T? HERBS AS MEDICINE

Herbs are another subset of functional foods because they have the ability to enhance our health. Herbs have been used medicinally for thousands of years, and their medicinal power has also been proven in clinical studies. However, along with the evolution of Western medicine, and its emphasis on pharmaceutical management of illness and disease came diminished awareness of the power of herbs.

We could write yet another book on their power, but for purpose of brevity, we will simply highlight some of the most widely accepted herbs, which have been scientifically studied.

Garlic is one of nature's wonders; it is a true super food, containing one of the broadest spectrums of antimicrobial action of any herb. In addition to its antiviral and antibacterial credentials, it has antifungal, antiparasitic, and antiprotozoan effectiveness. It can help reduce blood pressure, blood cholesterol, and triglyceride levels. Garlic's main active compound and the ingredient believed to stimulate the immune system, alliin (a sulphur compound which turns into the odorous allicin when the garlic is crushed or cut) reduces free radicals in the body, thus helping prevent colds and flu and perhaps even cancer.

Ginger is another wonder herb. Its most prominent attribute is perhaps its work in your gut. Ginger helps whatever ails you when it comes to stomach problems. Keep fresh ginger in your refrigerator, and cut off a piece if you have nausea or stomach discomfort. After removing the skin, chew on a piece (like spicy chewing gum) for fast relief, or make ginger tea.

Ginger has long been known as an efficient anti-inflammatory, antiflatulent, and antimicrobial. It relieves pain, reduces fever, lowers cholesterol, and soothes nerves, arthritis, and menstrual cramps. This is why the Chinese use it so extensively in their food and traditional medicine.

By raising body heat, ginger eliminates toxins associated with colds, and by stimulating circulation of blood in the pelvis, it helps relieve menstrual cramps. It can even reduce the painful effects of arthritis, and if applied directly on the chest or abdomen, it can relieve lung congestion, gas, and nausea.

Dandelion is another amazing herb, containing vitamins C and A, calcium, and more iron than spinach. Its distinguishing feature is its ability to act like a diuretic without depleting the body of potassium, like most other diuretics. This is because it is a source of potassium. Its ability to eliminate water helps the body get rid of harmful acids that accumulate during inflammation.

Milk thistle, also known as Our Lady's Thistle, is known for its ability to rehabilitate the liver. Because the liver is one of the most active and critical organs for detoxifying waste, this herb is one of the most important for use in detoxification. For example, liver poisoning from harmful chemicals, and less-serious problems such as poor digestion and liver function, experience positive effects and even cures through the use of milk thistle.

Milk thistle also influences weight loss through an antioxidant known as silymarin. This active compound protects the liver from free radicals and prevents toxins from entering the liver cells, which then allows it to regenerate properly. Problems such as cirrhosis, jaundice, and hepatitis, as well as damage from alcohol and drug abuse, are positively influenced by this herb.

Aloe vera was known in ancient Egypt as the "plant of immortality" and has a long history of being used to treat wounds, sun burn, psoriasis, diabetes, asthma, epilepsy, baldness, dandruff, and osteoarthritis. Today, it is widely used for its anti-inflammatory, regenerative, antibacterial, antifungal, anticancer, antileukemic, and antimutagenic properties. Topical creams applied to the skin can relieve pain quickly and speed the healing process for irritations, abrasions, and burns. Aloe also improves digestion and can be taken internally to heal tissues in our bowels and lungs, as well as mouth and stomach ulcers.

It is not known exactly which substances in aloe are responsible for its healing properties, but studies suggest that certain proteins in its composition may stimulate the immune system to produce more lymphocytes, the killer cells that help fight infections and tumors. Perhaps the most stunning of all its feats (for women who look for noninvasive ways to ward off time) is its ability to help stimulate synthesis of collagen in the skin, thus helping restore skin cells and prevent skin aging.

Ginseng: No list of herbs would be complete without ginseng, considered in Asian cultures as the ultimate elixir that can prolong life, increase resistance, prevent potency declines, and increase general vitality. These qualities are due to the herb's adaptogenic properties (a substance which enhances the body's ability to resist a stressor), which help regenerate and restore the body cells to a healthy state. It is considered by some to be a "super herb", one that fights inflammation, aging, oxidants, and cancer.

Due to its oxygenation properties, ginseng stimulates brain and physical activity, facilitates metabolism, strengthens the immune system, lowers cholesterol, controls blood sugar, and normalizes blood pressure. For men, ginseng's notoriety comes from its ability to help overcome erectile dysfunction as well as its antistress and antifatigue properties. For women, it helps with menopause symptoms.

Licorice is considered a superior balancing and harmonizing remedy, displaying strong anti-inflammatory, antiviral, and hormone-balancing properties. It is efficient in fighting inflammation, and it can restore general hormonal balance because of its active ingredient, glycyrrhizin. This compound gives the herb its characteristic flavor and can prolong the life of the cortisol (hormone) in the blood, thereby reducing the inflammation of bronchitis and sore throat.

Studies also show that licorice can effectively heal stomach ulcers by restoring the lining and mucous-secreting cells. Best of all, licorice root can be chewed as candies (it is also available in dried or powdered forms in capsules, tablets, and liquid extracts).

The power of spices, herbs, micronutrients and functional foods is one of the most underused weapons you have at your disposal to defend against the onslaught of toxins that can lead to degenerative diseases like cancer and arterial sclerosis (coronary artery disease characterized by thickening and hardening of the arteries' vessel walls resulting in sub-optimal blood flow to the heart). These powerful micronutrients not only provide beneficial chemicals that block various hormone actions and metabolic pathways associated with the development of cancer and heart disease, but they provide chemicals that stimulate protective enzymes.

This book has only scratched the surface of their importance. If you choose to live a longer, healthier and more satisfying life, incorporate micronutrients, phytonutrients, and functional foods with lots of color into your fuel stockpile for high-performance health.

As you navigate your health journey, learn more about which foods serve you, and incorporate as many as you can into your eating program. The following chart lists sources of phytochemicals found in functional foods and a summary of their potential benefits.

FUNCTIONAL FOODS WITH WELL-DOCUMENTED RESEARCH SUPPORTING THEIR BENEFITS

Functional Component	Potential Health Benefits, Low-Density Lipoprotein (LDL)	Food Source	Recommended Amount if Available
Beta-glucan (a soluble fiber)	Lower total blood cholesterol Lower LDL cholesterol	**Oats, oat bran, whole oat products**	3 grams per day
Catechins	May reduce risk of cancer; including gastric and esophageal May reduce risk of heart attack	**Green or black tea**	At least 3 cups per day

Isothiocya-nates	Lower risk of cancer	Broccoli, kale, and other cruciferous vegetables	At least 5 servings per week
Lycopene	Lower risk of cancer including prostate	Tomato and tomato products Cooking makes lycopene more bio-available	
Omega-3 fatty acids- DHA/ EPA	Lower risk of cardiovascular disease by lowering blood triglyceride levels	Cold-water fish and marine oils, including tuna, salmon, sardines, and mackerel	6 ounces fish per week
Organosulfur compounds	May inhibit platelet aggregation Lower total cholesterol Lower LDL cholesterol, triglycerides	Garlic	1 clove per day
Polyphenolic compounds	May lower risk of cardiovascular disease	Red and purple grapes, purple grape juice, red wine, peanuts	

Prebiotics (Fructoligo-saccharides, Insulin, polydextrose)	Support normal, healthy intestinal microflora	Jerusalem artichokes, chicory root, bananas, garlic, onions, whole grains	
Probiotics	Improve GI health	Fermented dairy products (yogurt/kefir)	
Soy Protein	May reduce risk of coronary heart disease Modest effect on lowering LDL cholesterol	Miso, tempeh, tofu, endamame (green soybeans)	50 grams per day

REFERENCES:

Vegetarian Nutrition, a dietetic practice group of the American Dietetic Association, 1998

Today's Dietitian, January 1999

IDEA Health and Fitness Source, February 1999

Linus Pauling Institute at Oregon State University

American Heart Association website

http://www.mckinley.illinois.edu/handouts/phytochemicals.htm

THE BIG THREE MACRONUTRIENTS

The big three macronutrients are carbohydrates, proteins, and fats.

You need all three categories, but the proportion from each group remains hotly contested. The USDA reissued its 1992 "food pyramid" in 2005 (it became "MyPyramid") and again in 2011 ("MyPlate") to reflect the proportions of foods you should include in your daily food program, but we believe that the generic prescription does not take into account bio-individuality and that you can assess the foods that match your individual needs. We also feel that the food pyramid does not distinguish between quality food fuel and food poison, so be aware of the differences in nutrient quality in your pursuit of an HP lifestyle program.

MACRONUTRIENT #1: CARBOHYDRATES

Do you want your body to drive like a Ferrari or an old Ford pickup? You can treat your only "vehicle" in this life like an expensive sports car that requires the highest quality maintenance and give it high-quality fuel, or you can give it low grade fuel and end up with a broken-down jalopy that needs constant repair. If you change one thing in your life, pay attention to the quality of your fuel. Not all fuel is good quality, and if you want to attain or sustain high performance, you need high-quality fuel. High-quality fuel for the body's engine is the same high-octane fuel you use for the brain: complex carbohydrates.

- Vegetables: Look for color
- Fruits: All kinds, all colors
- Legumes: Lentils, peas, and beans like kidney, pinto, black, and soy

- Whole grains: Drop white, refined grains from your diet; they lose their nutrients in processing

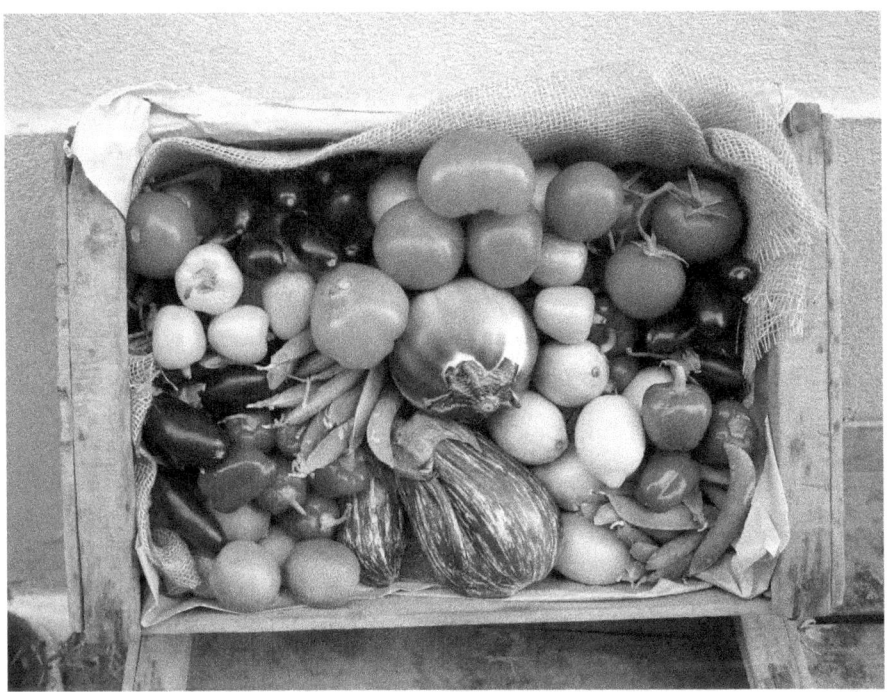

VEGETABLES: A CARB CATEGORY UNTO ITSELF

Have you heard the expression "you can never be too rich or too thin"? We tailor it to reflect our views on nutrition. "You can never be too healthy or have too many vegetables."

Vegetables contain varying amounts of the big three classic macronutrients, including protein and essential fatty acids. They are also key sources of fiber and prebiotics (non-digestable food that promotes good intestinal health), both essential for superior health and high performance.

However, their most notable attribute is not their macronutrient value but their micronutrient portfolio. Vegetables are one of two main sources for dense amounts of micronutrients, the sought-after antioxidant vitamins and minerals that we just spoke about. They are among the "super foods" in your fuel and energy arsenal because they contain vast amounts of micronutrients perfectly packaged in balanced doses for your needs.

Vegetables are a category unto themselves because they contain the other category of micronutrients we just talked about, the molecules called phytonutrients. If you wondered why healthy people are always pushing vegetables, you need wonder no longer. The importance of vegetables is so great that if we had to single out another game changer in the quest for high performance (after high-quality water), it would be "eat your vegetables and lots of them." This will ensure that you get the correct amounts of high-powered phytonutrients.

Only 10 percent of the US population consumes the five servings of fruits and vegetables recommended by the National Institutes of Health (NIH). *Most people go through the day without eating one serving.* Micronutrients are nonexistent in fast foods, overly processed food, and junk food. These processed foods instead contain vast amounts of refined sugar, which is not only devoid of micronutrients but is responsible for factors that suppress the immune system.[74]

Vegetables are *the* source of dense, immune-building, disease-preventing, performance-enhancing micronutrients, so they should make the biggest percentage of your daily food intake.

FRUITS FOR YOUR SWEET TOOTH: COLOR YOUR WORLD

Although fruits and vegetables contain many of the same nutrients (micronutrients and phytonutrients), fruits are generally much higher in carbohydrates, which is why we consider vegetables a separate class.

Similar to their high-quality vegetable counterpart, fruits are packed with antioxidants, phytochemicals, and essential minerals and vitamins.

They contain amazing, potent nutrients that give your body all kinds of health benefits including protection against cancer and cell damage.

The following list describes ten super fruits that build immunity, attack free radicals, and give high-quality energy. It is not a definitive list, as every nutritionist has his or her favorites.

1) **Berries**. Blueberries, strawberries, raspberries, goji, and acai. Berries contain a compound called **ellagic acid**, which is believed to help prevent cellular changes that can lead to cancer. The highest level of ellagic acid is found in raspberries. According to Gary D. Stoner, PhD, director of the cancer chemoprevention program at Ohio State University Comprehensive Cancer Center, ellagic acid is a powerful antioxidant, which "may help fight cancer on several fronts by reducing the damage caused by free radicals.... It also detoxifies carcinogens."[75]

Although all berries have high antioxidant values, blueberries and acai (from Brazil) are at the top of the list. Acai has **antioxidants** that combat premature aging, and it is packed with amino and essential fatty acids. Its unique combination of monounsaturated fats, dietary fiber, and phytosterols help promote cardiovascular and digestive health.

2) **Apple**. Always a symbol of health and vitality. Studies show that apples can help reduce the risk of heart disease. In laboratory research, they have stopping power against cancer cells. Much of the apple's healing power is in its skin, which contains large amounts of a compound called **quercetin**, an antioxidant that helps prevent oxygen molecules from damaging

cells that can inhibit the growth of tumors and prevent cancer from spreading.

3) **Cantaloupe.** A rich source of **potassium, antioxidants, vitamin C, and beta-carotene.** The powerful combination provides health benefits that include lowering blood pressure and cholesterol, reducing the risk of heart disease and cancer, and preventing cataracts. Potassium not only helps **lower blood pressure by helping eliminate excess sodium,** but it may help keep low-density lipoprotein (LDL) cholesterol from undergoing the chemical changes that cause it to stick to artery walls.

4) **Grapefruit.** These yellow and pink citrus balls relieve cold symptoms and prevent cancer, heart disease, and stroke. Grapefruits not only contain vitamin C, but they also contain other potent antioxidants that help reduce cold symptoms and decrease the risks of heart disease and cancer: **lycopene, limonoids, and naringin.**

   Lycopene, also found in sweet red peppers and tomatoes, is a free-radical scavenger, and **limonoids** have been shown to have anticancer properties; they increase the level of certain enzymes that help detoxify cancer-causing agents. **Naringin** has been shown to stop the growth of some kinds of breast cancer.

5) **Pear.** They fight cholesterol, improve memory and alertness, and keep bones strong. Pears contain a type of dietary fiber

called **lignin** that is effective for lowering cholesterol. Lignin, an insoluble fiber, helps usher cholesterol out of the body by acting like a type of Velcro, trapping cholesterol molecules in the intestine, before they get absorbed into the blood stream. Pears contain **pectin**, a soluble fiber that also binds with cholesterol and removes it, and pears contain **boron**, a mineral that plays an important role in keeping bones strong.

6) **Lemon and lime.** They prevent cancer and heart disease, help heal cuts and bruises, and prevent scurvy. We all know that vitamin C is a powerful antioxidant, but citrus fruits have more than just C. They also contain compounds called **limonin** and **limonene**, which appear to help block some of the cellular changes that can lead to cancer. **Limonene** is found primarily in the skin (or zest) of the fruit and has been shown to increase the activity of proteins that help eliminate estradiol, a naturally occurring hormone linked to breast cancer. **Limonene** also increases the level of enzymes in the liver, the major workhorse for detoxifying and removing cancer-causing chemicals.

7) **Pineapple.** These sweet and juicy tropical fruits are packed with vitamins, like vitamin A, vitamin C. They also have minerals like calcium, phosphorus and manganese, all of which help improve digestion, keep bones strong, and lower risk of cancer and heart disease. Most of us know that calcium is needed to keep bones strong; we also know that it must have magnesium to be properly absorbed. What we know less about is the formidable property of manganese.

Manganese helps make collagen, a tough, fibrous protein that can help build connective tissues like bone, skin, tendons, and cartilage. Research shows that people deficient in manganese develop bone problems similar to osteoporosis.

The phytochemical in pineapple is **bromelain**, an enzyme that helps digestion by breaking down proteins. Although not as rich in vitamin C as oranges or grapefruits, pineapples are packed with this vitamin (24 milligrams or 40 percent of RDA).

According to the NIH, bromelain is effective in reducing swelling (inflammation) of the nose and sinuses after surgery and injury. It is used for hay fever, treating bowel conditions that include swelling and ulcers, and removing dead and damaged tissue after a burn.

8) **Pomegranate.** This is an antioxidant powerhouse. Some studies suggest that the juice from pomegranates contain almost three times the total antioxidants in green tea and red wine. They also contain **polyphenols, tannins, and anthocyanins,** which can lower the risk of cancer, Alzheimer's disease, and premature aging. They help clear the arteries of plaque, which helps prevent heart disease and lowers blood pressure and the risk of stroke.[76]

9) **Kiwi.** An amazing weapon against cancer is this odd furry skinned green fruit. Kiwi has **phytonutrients, folic acid, fiber, vitamins C and E, zinc, calcium, magnesium,**

chromium, copper, iron, and potassium. Its phytonutrients help repair damage to DNA, the vitamins help with iron absorption and immunity, and the minerals enhance energy level and maintain the proper fluid balance.

Its antimutagenic component helps prevent the mutations of genes that initiate the cancer process. Scientists attribute this health benefit to the presence of **glutathione.**

Another phytochemical in kiwi, **lutein,** has been linked to the prevention of prostate and lung cancer. Kiwi contains **inositol,** a sugar alcohol (naturally occurring) that may play a positive role in regulating diabetes. Inositol helps facilitate responses to hormones and neurotransmitters, acting like a second messenger in the cell-signalling process.

10)   **Noni.** Although Noni is not often eaten as a fruit because of its bland taste and unpleasant smell, and its juice has probably one of the least appealing fruit flavors, its ability to provide protection against the development of cancer, protect the liver, relieve pain, and *reduce the amount of joint destruction caused by inflammation from arthritis* puts it into the top ten of the super fruit list. The high level of antioxidants in noni juice also boosts your immune system.

According to a study reported in the December 2001 issue of *Annals of the New York Academy of Sciences*, noni juice prevented the formation of cancer cells, and its extract had **antitumor properties.** Clearly, noni's antioxidant properties outweigh its less appealing taste, so drink it in shots if you want to reap the rewards of its health benefits.

LEGUMES: COMPLEX, ENERGY-PACKED CARBOHYDRATES

Legumes are another amazing category of complex carbohydrates to integrate into your weekly food program.

Legumes are beans and lentils; here is the short list:

- Black beans (also referred to as black turtle beans)
- Garbanzo beans (also referred to as chick peas)
- Kidney beans
- Lentils
- Lima beans
- Navy beans (also referred to as white beans)
- Peas
- Pinto beans
- Soybeans

GREAT NUTRITION IN SMALL PACKAGES

Legumes can help prevent diabetes and heart disease (they lower cholesterol) and cancer. They can help reduce cravings for sugar, therefore reducing the accumulation of fat leading to obesity, and they help prevent metabolic syndrome.[77]

They are inexpensive and packed with nutrition, including protein, calcium, vitamins, and minerals, and when cooked right, they can convert carnivores into fans.

Exactly how legumes provide such outstanding health benefits can be explained by how they are metabolized and their high micronutrient value.

Legumes provide slow-releasing energy and tons of high-quality nutrients without causing the pancreas to flood the body with insulin (like white carbs do). Eating legumes in place of fast-burning starch and refined carbs prevents the pancreas from releasing large amounts of insulin. Specifically, the pancreas produces only a certain amount of insulin, and repeated over-consumption of refined starches eventually depletes the pancreas, causing disruption of insulin production.[78] When legumes are eaten in place of refined carbs, your body does not overproduce insulin, which in turn helps to maintain healthy blood sugar levels and prevent type 2 diabetes.

A research team at the University of Queensland in Australia also identified a compound that reduces cancer risk and may help with cancer treatment.[79]

Last but not least, legumes, which have no cholesterol, help reduce cholesterol levels in the blood, thereby reducing or eliminating the risk of heart disease.

On the nutrition scale, legumes are powerful sources of antioxidants and are not only a good source of protein and energy, but they also provide many essential vitamins, minerals, and dietary fiber. They contain folate, manganese, magnesium, vitamin B1, phosphorus, iron, potassium, copper, and magnesium. Soybeans contain vitamin K and omega 3 fatty acids.

When you think of getting high-quality carbs, consider the benefits of lentils and beans, and you will rev up your energy engine and boost your immune defenses.

Now, just a quick review of the other complex carbs that we talked about as high quality fuel for the brain and body: whole grains.

WHOLE GRAINS: SMOKELESS FUEL FOR YOUR ENERGY ENGINE

Whole grains are a great source of fuel because they are high in fiber, which can help keep your intestinal health in good shape. Fibers are the brooms in your digestive system; they attach easily to the molecules and move them through the digestive tract. They have moderate levels of protein, and they are low in fat. Examples include millet, oats, wheat germ, barley, wild rice, brown rice, buckwheat, oat bran, cornmeal, and amaranth. If some of these grains are unfamiliar, ask for them in your supermarket or go to a specialty store that carries products made with whole grains. Any product made from whole grain is a complex carbohydrate: whole grain bread, bagels, pasta, macaroni, and some breakfast cereals. Be sure that the product is not loaded with sugar so that you can maximize the nutrient value.[80]

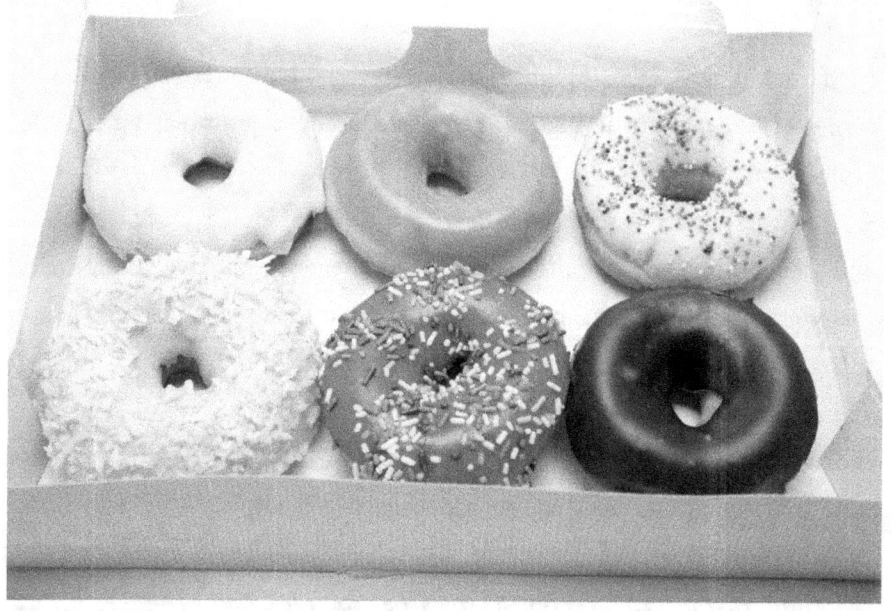

WHAT TO AVOID

Carbohydrates are your basic energy fuel supply, but not all carbs are good. Now that you know where to go for high-quality carbs, let's review where not to go.

- Starches: Pasta and bread (unless made with whole grain)
- Refined sugars, especially food with high fructose corn syrup
- Refined grains
- Processed food (chips, cookies, food in packages)
- Fast food
- **Alcohol**

All carbs provide the body with energy and the ability to store fat for days when food is in short supply (not a common phenomenon in the West, yet our bodies still retain this function). However, all carbs are converted to fat when you consume more than you need.

This point is important for those who think that cutting back on fat helps you lose weight. Products that are low in fat are usually high in sugar. This sugar will convert to fat and be stored because the body does not need it, but that's not the only problem with low-fat foods. When you don't have high-quality fats as fuel in your engine, your body is not satiated, and the hormones that tell you when you are hungry keep turning "on." Fat makes you feel full. Without them, you miss out on an important energy supply, and you get hungrier, faster.

If you want to lose weight, remember that refined sugars hidden in packaged goods and low-fat foods are your arch enemies, and good fats, your allies, help you maintain a healthy weight.

CLARIFICATION ABOUT SUGARS: AVOID SIMPLE SUGARS

Some people believe that simple sugars, defined as the simplest group of sugar (like sucrose or fructose), do not hydrolyse and result in faster blood sugar spikes than complex sugars. For example, the sugar you put in your coffee, and the sugar used in cakes, packaged foods, soda, fruit juice, honey, and sweets of all kinds, is simple sugar.

Why avoid these sugars? Simple sugars are quick energy sources, but they do not supply any other nutrients or fiber. *They are energy thieves.*

Most of the chips, crackers, and food in a package are filled with sugar in order to taste good. These are high in sugar but completely devoid of fiber. Because fiber makes you feel full, you get hungry faster and eat more. You take in less nutrients, less fiber, and more sugar, so you eat more and more. You get the picture. According to data from the National Health and Nutrition Examination Survey (2009-2010), more than 2 in 3 adults is considered to be overweight or obese. Welcome to the United States of Obesity, now at a record high and considered an epidemic in both children and adults.

Let's look again at complex sugars and why it is so important to include more of these carbs in your daily diet.

Complex sugars are found in fiber, whole-grain foods, raw vegetables and fruits (especially the seeds and skins), legumes, nuts, and seeds. They are called complex because the body needs to deconstruct them, metabolically speaking, and this process gives slow-releasing, sustainable energy.

Starches like bread, cereal, potatoes, pasta, and rice also have complex molecular structures, but they are broken down quickly and therefore act like simple sugars. You get rapid increases in insulin levels, which is not good for blood sugar balance.[81]

Conversely, not all simple sugars result in faster blood sugar spikes. Fructose, for example, is a simple sugar that does not trigger a rapid increase in blood sugar or insulin levels. Fructose, a good simple sugar, is found in milk and fruits. You get the sweetness and energy but not the "sugar high," because fructose is broken down differently from sucrose. Fruits, your allies in health, are also your allies in weight management, because they contain lots of fiber, and fiber helps maintain healthy intestines (the "broom effect"). They are a high-quality glucose fuel for the brain, a sugar hit for your sweet tooth, and contain high levels of phytochemicals that help reduce your appetite, thereby helping you to control weight.[82]

Finding good carbs is not usually a problem, but keeping bad carbs out of your food program is tricky. The world will surround you with temptations of inferior quality. The trick is to actively make choices that support your strategy for maintaining your high-end vehicle and quest for high performance. Finding breads, pastas, and sweets made with whole grains is a challenge, and converting your sweet tooth to a higher standard of pleasure will take ingenuity and patience. Choose sweets made with whole grains, raw organic sugar, or simply fruit.

High-quality carbs are found in the fruit and vegetable corners of the market where you shop, but high-quality grains are usually in small number or nonexistent unless you shop at an organic food shop or store that specialises in natural foods (like Whole Foods). The key to executing an HP eating plan is shopping at stores where you can find the high-quality foods you need and stores where you have multiple options. Getting used to switching from low quality, high refined sugar carbs is not always easy; this is why you will need a high dose of tenacity, commitment, and imagination.

Start slowly swapping out bad carbs. Think of them as energy bandits; they rob you of energy and keep you on a treadmill of sugar, stimulants, and stress. Good carbs are high-quality fuel for your energy batteries. When you are feeling hungry (an indication of low blood sugar), reach for fruit, seeds, nuts, or a whole-grain cracker that has the slower burning carbs. Check the sugar and trans fat or hydrogenated fat content in anything that comes in a package. When you must have something sweet, try dark chocolate, cookies made with whole grains, and strawberries with homemade whip cream. Slowly but surely, you will find alternatives for your standard go-to sweets.

Carbohydrates can energize the brain when eaten in moderation, or they can have a tranquillizing effect if eaten in excess. The body requires a specific level of glucose in the bloodstream to function correctly (just like it needs to maintain a temperature of 98.6 degrees). That level is two teaspoons of glucose for eight pints of blood. When you eat an excess of sweet foods, blood sugar goes out of balance, and the body struggles to return to a safe level. It will use vital resources that the cells need, making you tired and irritable.

Complex carbs are the highest quality fuel for your brain and body metabolism because they are broken down slowly, and digestion releases the glucose into the bloodstream at a steady pace. They are the type of food our ancestors ate, not the quick sugar fixes that are damaging to your metabolism and energy engine.

There is accumulating evidence that sugar reduces the immune system's ability to fight infection. It can cause mineral problems, like copper deficiency, and it can produce an acidic digestive tract. High sugar consumption can lead to alcoholism, premature aging of organs, high blood pressure, heart disease, arteriosclerosis, and type 2 diabetes.[83]

Now that you know better, be on the lookout for energy bandits, the "white enemy" in the food supply—refined sugar and flour found in cakes, crackers, pasta, bread, and packaged foods. Stick with high-quality fuel: complex carbs in whole grains, legumes, vegetables, and fruits. We may sound like a broken record, but we cannot emphasize this enough.

ALCOHOL: THIS ANTI-NUTRIENT IS YOUR BRAIN'S ENEMY

Alcohol is an anti-nutrient because it depletes almost every vitamin in your body. It disturbs your blood sugar balance, one of the key balances for health and HP. The list of vitamins and minerals it depletes is long: vitamins A, B1, B2, B6, B12, C, D, E, folic acid, calcium, magnesium, potassium, zinc, and selenium. It robs you of amino acids, like tryptophan, taurine, and glutathione, as well as the essential fats like omega 3 and 6 that you need for a high-functioning brain.

Put simply by Patrick Holford, "Alcohol is the brain's worst enemy... (because it) pickles your brain."[84]

The pickling, according to Holford, happens because the brain is incapable of detoxifying alcohol (hence the "high"). Once the liver's capacity is exceeded, the alcohol disrupts the brain's signals, so you feel giddy as your cognitive abilities erode. The weakening of brain signals also begins to erode your ability to remember things. This is good for anyone seeking to temporarily remove anxieties but not good in the long term for high performance.

Alcohol dissolves the important fatty acids in brain cells and even replaces good fat with bad fat by blocking the conversion of fats into DHA and prostaglandins. This is also why you see diminished mental abilities and impairment of motor skills.

Dr. Amen lectures frequently on the dangers of alcohol because its impact on the brain is evident in his brain-imaging studies. With a library of research containing over seventy thousand SPECT brain scans (Single-Photon Emission Computed Tomography, designed to track blood flow in the brain and show areas of high and low activity), Amen proves that alcohol creates dark crevasses and cavities, similar to those found in patients with Alzheimer's disease. These brains are not just those of alcoholics but also of people who consume alcohol regularly.[85]

Forget about the doctor's advice about two glasses of wine (unless it's two or three glasses a week), and stick with the advice of two apples a day. Alcohol creates problems for your brain. Use as little as possible, and if you must indulge, make sure it's on a special occasions and a moderate amount. If it is part of your daily fuel intake, you will destroy the nutrients and construction materials that you need for an HP lifestyle.

MACRONUTRIENT #2: FATS

Since we discussed Fats and their role in contributing to higher brain function, let's expand upon some of the basic information.

Fats are vital to health—the good fats, that is. The brain is two-thirds fat, every cell membrane in the body contains fat in the form of phospholipids, and the element of neurotransmission in the brain (the myelin sheath) depends on having the correct amount of essential fatty acids derived from good fats.

Many of us have been taught that fats are fattening (the "fat makes us fat theory:" seems to make sense) and that they also raise cholesterol and should be avoided at all costs. Wrong.

While low-fat options have exploded, so have our waistlines. Clearly, the low-fat food craze has not worked out as planned. We were led down the wrong path. The vast proliferation of low-fat foods in supermarkets seemed to offer an endless array of guilt-free options—baked potato chips, fat-free ice cream, low-fat cookies, cakes, low-fat, guilt-free everything. There was an implicit promise: cut out fat, and you can eat your favorite foods and not gain weight (the "no-fat-in = no-fat-on" theory). Oops. Wrong again.

These foods and low-fat diets have not only *not* delivered on the promise to keep us trim, they have sabotaged our ability to maintain good health. So what is wrong with this picture? Why don't low-fat options give us guilt-free pleasure without the added inches on our hips?

Here is the skinny on fat. Despite what you have been told, fat isn't the bad guy. The bad fats, those excess, saturated fats combined with fried carbs and trans fats, are guilty as charged for weight gain, clogged arteries, and high cholesterol.

Fats are vital to health, and you need fats in your diet. However, make smart choices. Bad fats can make you fat, whereas the good fats keep you satiated and help your body build and repair cells. They play a huge role in helping manage moods, they keep brain synapses firing and joints flexible, and they help you control weight.

The answer isn't to cut out fats but rather learning which fats are part of a health regimen and which fats clog the brain and arteries. Remember that bad carbs convert to fat when they are not used for energy, so keep this in mind when choosing a low-fat, high-sugar food that is essentially making you fat.

Let's get the fat story straight. There are **four** main types of fat: saturated, monounsaturated, polyunsaturated (all naturally occurring), and trans (manufactured by adding one hydrogen molecule).

Since trans fats are more often than not artificial and processed, have no nutritional value, and are dangerous (because they cannot be digested properly and raise bad cholesterol-LDL- while lowering good cholesterol-HDL), they should be avoided entirely. A small percentage of what you ingest is naturally occurring in food, and we are not referring to this form because it can be digested.

Trans fats are produced by a process called *hydrogenation*, which increases their shelf life and flavor stability. Because these fats are commonly used in packaged food products, including vegetable shortening; cereals; candies; snack foods like cookies, granola bars, and chips; as well as salad dressings, margarine, crackers (even ones that seem healthy like Nabisco Wheat Thins), and fried foods (to name a few), you need to pay close attention to the labels on the food you buy. Lastly, beware of trans fats masquerading as hydrogenated and partially hydrogenated fats.

Let's get to the remaining three fats. According to the 2005 Dietary Guidelines for Americans, 20–35 percent of total calories should come from monounsaturated and polyunsaturated fats, with less than 10 percent from saturated fats. The unfortunate fact is that the modern diet is much higher in saturated and trans fat and contains much less of the good fats.

The good fats are polyunsaturated (*poly* means very) and monounsaturated. These fats, listed below, are considered the "good fats" because they are good for your heart, cholesterol, and overall health. Keep in mind that the essential fats omega-3 and omega-6, which have to be obtained through the food you eat, are polyunsaturated.

GOOD FATS	
▪ Olive oil	▪ Soybean oil
▪ Canola oil	▪ Corn oil
▪ Sunflower oil	▪ Safflower oil
▪ Peanut oil	▪ Walnuts
▪ Sesame oil	▪ Sunflower, sesame, and pumpkin seeds Flaxseed
▪ Avocados	
▪ Olives	▪ Fatty fish (salmon, tuna, mackerel, herring, trout, sardines)
▪ Nuts (almonds, peanuts, macadamia, hazel, pecans, cashews)	
	▪ Soymilk
▪ Peanut butter	▪ Tofu

The best sources for good fats are nuts, natural peanut butter, vegetable oils, avocados, seeds, and fish.

Nuts are highest in monounsaturated fat and contain some polyunsaturated fat. Natural peanut butter is a great source of monounsaturated fat, but buyers beware: avoid processed peanut butter unless you buy it in a "green" store with organic produce. The processed kind can have added sugar and hydrogenated oils (trans fats).

Everyone knows about olive oil; it is one of the best sources of monounsaturated fats and is lower in saturated fat than other oils, but other oils are also rich sources of good fat.

What about those fantastic avocados? We cringe when we hear people say that they avoid avocados because they have so much fat. This is exactly the problem with our perceptions about fat. That same person will turn around and eat a bowl of potato chips or order a hamburger with highly saturated fats, along with French fries that have been deep fried (with no guarantee that the frying oil was not rancid). Avocados are a super, natural food and great with olive oil and lemon or in a guacamole.

Seeds contain oils that are lower in saturated fat and higher in unsaturated fats. Sesame and pumpkin seeds contain some of the highest concentrations of monounsaturated fat, so incorporate them into your salads or alone as a snack. Pumpkin and sunflower seeds are great to keep in a Ziploc bag to snack on in the office or while running errands.[86]

The best sources for omega-3 are fatty fish like salmon, herring, mackerel, anchovies, and sardines. You can also get high-quality, cold-water fish oil supplements.

Some people avoid fish because they are concerned about mercury and other possible toxins. Most experts agree that the benefits of eating two servings a week of cold-water fatty fish outweigh the risks. If you are still concerned, rotate your fish consumption. Stick with smaller fish like sardines and anchovies that tend to have smaller amounts of mercury. If you are a vegetarian or don't like fish, find a high-quality fish oil supplement, or get omega 3 by eating algae. Better yet, try hemp and hemp oil, pumpkin, pumpkin oil, flaxseeds, walnuts, and chia seeds.

Bad fats are guilty of making you fat, unhealthy, unhappy, and moody, and they can cause problems in your brain.

We have included a chart below of foods containing trans fat, and if you can't carry a copy of it in your wallet, remember that saturated and trans fats tend to be solid at room temperature (like a stick of margarine), and monounsaturated or polyunsaturated fats tend to be liquid. Although we are not dismissing saturated fats entirely as bad, we are pointing out that too much saturated fats in your diet (the recommended percentage is 10 percent of total fat), combined with other lifestyle factors, can adversely affect your health. The "villain" fat, trans fat, is unequivocally bad for your health, so keep it out of your diet entirely.

An excellent source of a good fat is coconut oil. Although it is a saturated fat, we consider it to be one of the good fats, as long as it is cold-pressed, organic coconut oil, which exists in both solid and liquid form, depending on the time of year.

THE EVIL FAT
Trans fat
■ Commercially baked pastries, cookies, doughnuts, muffins, cakes, pizza dough
■ Packaged snack food (crackers, microwave popcorn, chips)
■ Stick margarine
■ Vegetable shortening
■ Fast food
■ Fried food (French fries, fried chicken, chicken nuggets, breaded fish)
■ Frozen food
■ Candy bars
■ Cake mixes

MACRONUTRIENT #3: PROTEINS

Proteins are found in meats, poultry, and fish. They are also in beans, nuts, seeds and legumes, eggs, and dairy products like milk and cheese.

Proteins from animal sources contain all the amino acids you require nutritionally and are therefore considered complete proteins. Proteins from vegetable sources, on the other hand, are not complete and must be combined to give you a complete protein.

ENERGY, MOOD, AND BLOOD BALANCE DEPEND ON THEM

Proteins provide amino acids, which are the building materials for cells that help balance blood sugar. More importantly, the amino acids from protein provide the raw material you need to synthesize neurotransmitters, enzymes, hormones, and cells used for immunity.

Without them, the body cannot build and repair cells or manufacture the enzymes that call the shots in biochemical reactions. Your ability to fight infection is also compromised if you do not get the correct balance of amino acids from protein.

Proteins are also critical for balancing energy, and they can affect mood. L-tyrosine for example, an amino acid found in meat, poultry, fish, and tofu, is the precursor to dopamine, epinephrine, and norepinephrine, all of which are critical for balancing mood and energy. Keep in mind that stress and fatigue also use your supply of important vitamins and can deplete norepinephrine. Your body then needs more L-tyrosine to replenish it.

Another example is L-tryptophan, a building block for serotonin. You want an ample supply of this mood-regulating neurotransmitter. According to Dr. Amen, increasing intake of this amino acid, found in meat eggs, milk, soy, lentils, sesame, peanuts, pumpkin, and rice, can be helpful for some people in stabilizing mood and improving mental clarity and sleep.[87]

So, cutting to the chase, what foods should you be eating, and how much?

IF YOU LIKE MEAT, POULTRY, OR FISH

Our formula is simple. Maintain high-quality, lean protein intake from protein-rich foods like fish, skinless chicken and turkey, and lean beef; reduce your intake of red meats, unless the animal was raised on farms with grass feed (as in countries like Argentina); and go "organic" to reduce your intake of toxins (e.g., antibiotics are routinely fed to poultry and cattle). Fish are an especially good source of protein because you get both the nutrient value of omega 3 fats and protein. Incorporate as much protein as you can from beans, raw nuts, and high-protein grains and vegetables. This will help reduce your reliance on meat.

Animal protein is harder to digest than vegetable protein, and it puts a strain on your detoxification system when you eat too much of it. Many people today suffer from weak digestive systems. Animal proteins are higher in the food chain and therefore have more toxins than vegetable proteins, so increase your consumption of vegetable proteins in your quest for superior health.

When you do eat meat and poultry, make sure that it is free of hormones and antibiotics and raised free range to maximize the quality of the protein and reduce the toxins that your body must remove. Remember that vegetables, not meat, should constitute the biggest percentage of your daily food intake.

If you are a vegetarian, the formula is different. Not all proteins are created equal. Proteins from animal sources provide a complete slate of amino acids, whereas vegetable proteins (with a few exceptions, like tofu) must be combined. If you are vegetarian, watch for sources of complete proteins.

Let's elaborate. At least twenty amino acids are necessary for human nutrition, all of which are indispensable for superior health and immunity. Just like fats, some of these amino acids can be manufactured in the body (therefore termed "nonessential"), but others, referred to as "essential," must be obtained from food.

Still other nonessential amino acids are made from essential ones, so they are called "semi-essential." Once you learn which vegetables can be combined to give you a complete amino acid, you are set. Any combination of whole grain and legumes or peanut butter and whole wheat, or rice and beans, can give you a complete protein. *Keep in mind that complete proteins do not need to be obtained in the same meal; they can be eaten at different times during the day.*

If you want to give your brain a "clarity shot," forget the coffee, and try a high-powered green protein drink made from vegetable sources. Vegetable proteins from greens have all the amino acids you get from animal sources, without the toxins. A green drink will boost your attention and focus, whereas carbohydrates in donuts, bagels, and/or cereal will boost serotonin, which induces relaxation and drowsiness. When you are looking for a competitive advantage, clarity, and focus in your next business meeting, start your day with a high-powered, green drink juiced from dark-green leafy vegetables. Throw in apples and ginger for sweetness and spice.

THE VALUE OF HIGH-QUALITY WATER

Water is the most abundant nutrient in the body. It comprises two-thirds of your body's mass and is a vital component in all body functions. To give optimal benefit, water should have three qualities:

1) It should have a good pH (that is, it should be more alkaline and not acidic).

2) It should have an oxidation reduction potential (ORP), the component that allows it to reduce oxidation, which then reduces free-radical production.

3) It should have good filtration, reducing the toxins, chemicals, and bacteria that might get into your body.

Before the Industrial Revolution, water from springs, waterfalls, lakes, and wells was clean. Even rainwater was considered a good source of drinking water. This is no longer the case.

Water has its own intrinsic energy when it is not polluted with chemicals or combined with wastes that diminish its energy. Today, as rainwater falls through the atmosphere, it encounters pollution that encircles the earth, picking up smoke, dust, germs, lead, strontium 90[*], minerals, and a host of other chemicals.

Even wells can contain high levels of pollutants, because they are often close to chemical agriculture and livestock. Surface water combines with the residue of poison sprays, fertilizers, and animal excrement, which seep into the water table. A major toxin in farm wells is nitrate from farm chemicals, which converts into carcinogenic nitrites by heating, microbial action, or contact with certain metals. According to toxicology researchers, some of the chemicals present in well water are herbicides, defoliants, pesticides, and soil fumigants.

What about the water in our cities? According to federal water studies, "There is a 40 percent chance that the next water you drink will have passed through someone's sewer or an industrial conduit filled with wastes, poisons, and bacteria."[88]

---

[*] Strontium 90 is a radioactive metallic element that has entered the food chain through ingestion of contaminated foods and cow's milk. The primary source is from weapons testing fallout; however, radioactive releases from nuclear power plants (Fukushima and the 1986 Chernobyl accident) have also contaminated our food sources.

A trend in large American cities is recycling used water that is contaminated with bacteria, human excrement, and chemicals, cleaning it with chlorine, and adding sodium fluoride for tooth-decay prevention.

CHLORINATION

Once out of the tap, chlorine evaporates; many people draw chlorinated water and let it stand at least thirty minutes. Unfortunately, chlorine combines with any organic substance that may be present, and it forms chloroform, a cancer-causing chemical that does not evaporate.

Chlorine in drinking water also creates those pesky electrically charged molecules known as free radicals, which can cause damage to the blood vessels, resulting in plaque and arterial heart disease.

When chlorine is regularly ingested, it destroys vitamin E, and its presence is closely linked with vascular disease. It also destroys beneficial flora in the intestines. Chlorine itself is so hazardous on the surface of the body, that even the Environmental Protection Agency (EPA) has warned that prolonged swimming or bathing in chlorinated water contributes to skin cancer.

Let's take a closer look at why chlorine is such a dangerous environmental toxin. Chlorine's danger stems from its ability to bind to organic matter and produce chemicals called organochlorines, almost all of which are foreign to nature. The majority of organochlorines are stable, which is to say that they do not break down in the environment for hundreds of years! Chlorine-based poisons tend to bio-accumulate over time, so they build up in the body fat of humans and other animals. When you know that this chemical is poisonous to your organs, destroying vitamins and intestinal flora, imagine the damage it can do over time if it accumulates and lingers in your cells.

According to research in Canada and the United States, 177 different organochlorines have been found in the fat, semen, blood, breath, and mother's milk of the population. Although each person can have a different tolerance for the organochlorines, contamination can trigger a wide range of health problems, including hormonal disruption, infertility, lowered sperm count, immune system suppression, learning disabilities, behavioral changes, and damage to the skin, liver, and kidneys.

FLUORIDATION

The sodium fluoride approved by the FDA in 1964 and used in the water supplies is a drug with insidious effects on health:

1) Fluorite, a naturally occurring compound of calcium and fluoride, is used as a tranquilizer in traditional Chinese medicine

2) Prozac, an antidepressant, is based on the fluoride molecule fluoxetine hydrochloride.

3) The original decay prevention tests with fluoride were carried out with *calcium fluoride*; however, it is not calcium fluoride but sodium fluoride and fluorosilicic acid that is added to city water supplies.

4) These chemicals are toxic by-products of the aluminium and fertilizer industries and are often highly contaminated with lead and arsenic.

5) The chemical by-products of aluminium and fertilizer companies were expensive to dispose of until cities were

persuaded to put them in the public water for tooth-decay prevention.

6) Until this time, the primary use of fluoride was as rat poison.

7) After approval for city water, the price of sodium fluoride shot up 1,000 percent.

8) As a result of research in Europe, fluoride treatment of water is illegal in Sweden, Denmark, and Holland. Germany and Belgium have discontinued fluoride experiments on humans, and France and Norway never found sufficient evidence to warrant water fluoridation.

9) Studies indicate that fluoride per se is one of nature's principal aging factors.[89]

10) A meta-analysis funded by the National Institutes of Health (NIH) and published by Harvard University concluded that children who live in areas with highly fluoridated water have "significantly lower" IQ scores than those who live in low fluoride areas.[90,91]

Here is a quick look at the impact of fluoride:

- It inhibits the proper functioning of the thyroid gland and all enzyme systems, making weight reduction more difficult.
- It damages the immune system and can lead to serious disorders like sclera derma, lupus, and forms of arthritis.[92]

OTHER CHEMICALS

A number of other chemicals are intentionally added by some water departments to stabilize the action of water and keep city pipes from rusting:

- Seventy thousand chemicals are now in commercial production, and the EPA has listed sixty thousand of them as potentially or definitely hazardous to human health.
- Three hundred million tons of waste are generated by industry annually, and the EPA estimates that 90 percent of this waste is improperly disposed, finding its way directly or indirectly into the air you breathe, the water you drink, and/or the soil in which you grow food.

What does all this mean? It means that drinking tap water is no longer an option.

We must be vigilant about the chemicals seeping into our water supply and into us. It affects the brain, thinking (remember that sodium fluoride is used as a sedative in Chinese medicine), and health.

Because it is unlikely that you can fix the city water supply where you live, filter your water to remove the majority of bacteria, mold, fluoride, chlorine, chloramines, heavy metals, and hormones.

An even better option, although somewhat controversial, is to install an alkaline water ionization filter in your home or office. This provides three benefits:

1) It provides alkaline pH water.

2) It provides ORP.

3) It provides filtered water.

These benefits enhance your immune system, give your cells more nourishment, and reduce or eliminate the toxins and residual chemicals found in city water. We highly recommend investing in better health with a water filter system that provides alkaline ionized water.[93]

Another option is to use activated charcoal filters, which can remove most of the wastes and other toxins that are not water soluble. The major water-soluble dangers are nitrates, nitrites, and sodium fluoride. If these chemicals are present, a filter can be useful if a) it has a strong filtering ability, b) it does not accumulate bacteria, and c) it is replaced as instructed when the filtering capacity is exhausted.

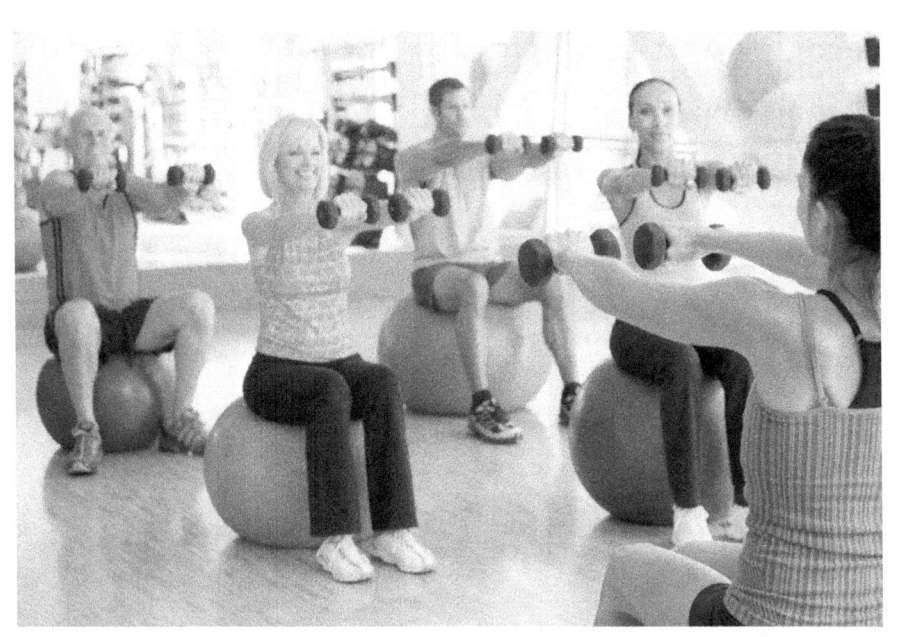

CHAPTER 7:

☆ ☆ ☆

ACTIVITY CREATES VITALITY

STEP 6: EXERCISE DAILY. PHYSICAL ACTIVITY (RESPIRATION AND PERSPIRATION) GENERATES VITALITY AND ENERGY, BUILDS STAMINA, AND IMPROVES BRAIN PERFORMANCE.

"Physical fitness is not only one of the most important keys to a healthy body, it is the basis of dynamic and creative intellectual activity." **—John F. Kennedy**

EXERCISE: THE ELIXIR FOR ENERGY, VITALITY, IMMUNITY

A few generations ago, most people were active. They worked hard physically in their daily chores and jobs. The conveniences of the modern world were not as available, so people walked more and sat less.

The world of our grandfathers and great- grandfathers had fewer escalators and cars and no remote controls. Take-out food was virtually nonexistent.

Today, we park as close as we can to the entrances of stores, lest we have to walk the length of a parking lot. Pushing buttons, touch-screen computers, delivery service, and take-out foods bring everything to us while we exert little or no physical effort to get them. We don't have to walk to a library to return a book; libraries are at the touch of a computer screen, a Google search away.

All of this relative inactivity has resulted in an overweight population in the US and most of the Westernized world. Compared to our ancestors, we are not only grossly overweight, but we also have functional problems like diabetes, heart disease, cancer.

This phenomenon is the result of five converging lifestyle changes: inactivity due to modern conveniences, workplace demands, recreational choices (sitting in front of computer screens for hours, for example), nutrient-poor diet (micronutrient starvation), and a toxic external and internal environment.

BENEFITS OF EXERCISE

Like it or not, your body was designed for physical activity.

If you want to have good health, avoid diseases, keep your immunity strong, maintain a good physical appearance, extend your life, and maintain higher levels of cognitive function, exercise is a basic requirement. Let's look at the benefits of exercise, which are in and of themselves motivating.

EXERCISE JUMPSTARTS NEUROGENESIS AND SLOWS BRAIN DECAY

Until the 1990s, conventional wisdom and scientists believed that we were born with a certain number of brain cells, but in the 1990s, researchers determined, during autopsies, that the human brain contained new neurons, especially in the area of the hippocampus, the region related to memory and certain types of learning.[94]

The creation of new neurons, or neurogenesis, was a major breakthrough in neuroscience. The discovery dispelled the long-standing belief that what we have in terms of brainpower is all we ever have.

For all of us who worried that brain cells were destroyed in our wanton youths, this is good news. The discovery that exercise can jumpstart neurogenesis means that we can reverse memory impairment and improve some cognitive functions by being active.

Exercise increases the formation of new brain cells, which means it can slow down and even reverse the brain's physical decay, the same as with muscles.

EXERCISE AMPLIFIES DETOXIFICATION

Exercise is essential for detoxification, one of the most important activities of your metabolism. Lack of exercise causes toxins to build up in your body, which upsets homeostasis. On the flip side, exercise improves the activity of liver detoxification. The act of moving speeds up the removal of toxins and waste materials from cells and increases blood flow, carrying nutrients to the cells more efficiently.

EXERCISE STRENGTHENS YOUR CARDIOVASCULAR SYSTEM

Exercise strengthens the cardiovascular system and can help lower blood pressure and cholesterol, which helps prevent heart attacks. According to the American Heart Association (AHA), regular physical activity helps you combat hardening of the arteries (atherosclerosis) by improving your heart's ability to pump and keeping your veins and arteries toned.

In general, your cardiovascular fitness is a measure of how efficiently your heart can circulate blood to your organs. The more physically fit you are, the more efficiently your circulatory system pumps blood to your organs, including your brain, a necessary health benefit for HP. Following the advice of the AHA, we recommend combining aerobic and resistance exercises for greatest cardiovascular benefit.[95]

EXERCISE IMPROVES OVERALL PHYSIOLOGY

Exercise stimulates numerous mechanisms, which in turn help improve overall physiology. It reduces the quantity of adipose tissue, which is the principal storage site of toxins, particularly carcinogenic toxins. It improves your hormonal balance by reducing the excess estrogens and testosterone that stimulate the growth of tumors.[96]

A consistent program of exercise increases your body temperature (sweating reduces toxins), restores lung power, and improves bone structure and muscle flexibility. Exercise gives your inner organs and systems a workout, which keeps them vital and helps them function better.

EXERCISE KEEPS YOU LOOKING AND FEELING YOUNGER, LONGER

According to Dr. Amen, in *"Use Your Brain to Change Your Age,"*[97] a recent study showed that after age sixty-five, one strong predictor of longevity is walking speed. Those who can still hoof it after age seventy-five have a better chance of living longer. An eighty-year-old man who clocks even one mile per hour has a 10 percent probability of reaching ninety, while a woman of the same age walking at that pace has a 23 percent greater chance.

Amen also points out that exercising thirty minutes a day, five times a week, slows your biological age. He cites research from the University of St. Andrews in Scotland that revealed that the signs of aging, like sagging skin under the chin and around the neck and jowls, are more pronounced in people who do not exercise. The tell-tale area around the forehead and eyes tends to fatten more in people who are inactive.

EXERCISE CHANGES YOUR BIOLOGICAL AGE

If you are up to date on research on aging, you have come across exciting studies that link longevity to the length of telomeres, which are the protective covering of chromosomes strands. Your telomeres control your aging. The shorter they are, the faster you age, and as you age, they shorten. Researchers also believe that the shorter your telomeres get, the higher your risk of age-related diseases like high blood pressure, mental decline, and cancer. The good news is that you can lengthen your telomeres with exercise, and you don't need a lot. Three hours a week will do the trick.[98]

Studies have been conducted over the last five to ten years that support this. The studies strengthen the conclusion that exercising regularly is likely to protect your telomere lengths, and that vigorous aerobic exercise keeps telomere lengths at youthful levels. If your goal is to maintain or improve upon the energy of your younger self, staying active pays off.[99]

EXERCISE HELPS BALANCE BLOOD SUGAR

Maintaining balanced blood sugar is one of the key metabolic markers for HP. Exercise reduces blood sugar levels, which in turn reduces the secretion of insulin and other hormones such as insulin-like growth factor (IGF), which contribute to inflammation. Although it is not fully understood why, scientists have studies that show that sedentary people are at increased risk of developing type 2 diabetes.

A study at the University of Missouri in 2011, conducted by John P. Thyfault, associate professor of nutrition and exercise physiology, among a group of healthy, active young adults, revealed that physical languor affected the body's ability to control blood sugar spikes. The study showed that after just three days of inactivity, the volunteers' blood sugar levels spiked after meals by about 26 percent compared to when they were exercising and moving more. Thyfault is quoted as saying that inactivity is dangerous when it becomes the body's default condition; "we hypothesize that, over time, inactivity creates the physiological conditions that produce chronic disease," like type 2 diabetes and heart disease, regardless of a person's weight or diet.[100]

EXERCISE HELPS REDUCE INFLAMMATION

According to various studies, physical exercise acts directly on reducing inflammatory response mechanisms called cytokines that are responsible for inflammation.[101]

EXERCISE IMPROVES THE IMMUNE SYSTEM

Exercise has a direct effect on the immune system and appears to play a major role in healing. According to Dr. Joseph Mercola, one of the leading proponents on fitness and strong immunity, "exercise is a critical component of good health, especially as you age."

- It helps improve your resistance to fight infections.
- It lowers your risk of cancer, heart disease and diabetes.
- It helps your brain work better, making you smarter.[102]

EXERCISE ELEVATES EMOTIONAL WELL-BEING

Studies also show that exercise has a positive impact on emotional and psychological well-being, elevating mood with the release of natural biochemicals like endorphins, and neurotransmitters. These chemicals create norepinephrine, dopamine, and serotonin, all of which elevate your mood.

EXERCISE REGULATES METABOLISM, MAKING WEIGHT MANAGEMENT MORE SUSTAINABLE

People who exercise regularly actually "program" their muscles' ability to burn fat more efficiently. This is partly because exercise allows the body to mobilize fatty acids from your fat deposits into your bloodstream, so that your metabolism becomes more of a fat-burning engine. The side benefits are that the exercise reduces your insulin resistance and triglycerides and increases your HDL levels of cholesterol (the good cholesterol). Exercising also decreases anger and hostility and reduces stress.

What about the "high" that people talk about? We've all heard of the state of mind that kicks in after twenty to thirty minutes of sustained jogging or "runner's high." It is true. This is exactly the effect that sustained exercise can have in the short term and long term. Endorphins, which get aroused with thirty minutes of exercise, attach to the same neuron receptors as opiates like morphine and heroin. This is why you get a boost in energy and emotional outlook when you exercise. After you get into having a steady dose of exercise, it will become something your body craves, like a natural drug.

The ability of physical activity to improve your mental state is so well documented that the Ministry of Health in the United Kingdom recommends exercise as a first intervention for depression, on par with chemical antidepressants.[103,104]

MOVE IT (YOUR BODY) OR LOSE IT (YOUR MIND): LACK OF EXERCISE SHRINKS THE BRAIN AND STOPS NEUROGENESIS

Because we are talking about HP and the things that enhance or diminish the primary resource for achieving it (the brain), it is helpful to know that you can stimulate neurogenesis via lifestyle and nutrition choices.

Studies show that mental stimulation, such as learning a new skill, a new language, crossword puzzles, and physical exercise improve brain function and protect it against cognitive decline. This is because the human brain is continually adapting and rewiring itself. Even in old age, you can grow new neurons if you remain active. Severe mental decline is usually caused by disease, whereas most age-related memory declines or losses in motor skills are the result of inactivity and lack of mental stimulation.

The old adage "use it or lose it" is based on scientific research. Some of this research was recently published in *The New York Times*.[105] According to the article, a team of researchers, led by Justin S. Rhodes, a psychology professor at the Beckman Institute for Advanced Science and Technology at the University of Illinois, conducted cognitive experiments with mice to track changes in their brain structures and determine the impact of exercise versus other controlled variables. Their results?

According to Rhodes, "Only one thing had mattered, and that's whether they had a running wheel." Based on the study, animals that exercised, whether or not they had any other enrichment in their cages, had healthier brains and performed significantly better on cognitive tests than the other mice. Animals that didn't exercise, no matter how enriched their world was in terms of living environment (stimulation from neon-hued balls, plastic tunnels, mirrors, and other kinds of pleasures and embellishments) did not improve their brainpower.

PREVENTING COGNITIVE DECLINE

A study by researchers at the Center for Hip Health and Mobility at Vancouver Coastal Health and the University of British Columbia demonstrated that exercise, particularly resistance training, altered the trajectory of cognitive decline among the elderly. The study was published in the April 23, 2012 edition of *Archives of Internal Medicine* and reviewed in *Science Daily*. According to the article, "The exercise program improved the executive cognitive process of selective attention and conflict resolution functions, as well as associative memory, which are robust predictors for conversion from mild cognitive impairment to dementia."

Although the principal investigator of the research, Teresa Liu-Ambrose, acknowledged the controversy surrounding the impact of exercise on the trajectory of cognitive impairment and decline, she argued that *the results of her study indicated a clear and convincing relationship.* "What our results show is that resistance training can indeed improve both your cognitive performance and your brain function. What is key is that the training will improve two processes that are highly sensitive to the effects of aging and neuro-degeneration-executive function and associative memory- functions which are often impaired in early stages of Alzheimer's disease."[106]

A PROTEIN THAT PROMOTES HEALTHY NEURONS

Brain-derived neurotrophic factor (BDNF) is a dream protein in your brain when you have an abundance of it. It has been researched and proven to promote the health of nerve cells in the brain. Specifically, it strengthens cells and axons and fortifies connections among the neurons, which in turn stimulates the process of neurogenesis. Scientists found that after workouts, most people display higher BDNF levels in their bloodstream.

In a Brazilian experiment, scientists found that elderly rats that ran for five minutes several days per week over a five-week period showed remarkable improvement in biochemical processes, particularly in their memory center, where the production of BDNF molecules had increased. The older animals that exercised even outperformed the younger rats on memory tests.[107]

A more convincing study conducted among pilots aged forty to sixty-five, and published in 2011 in *Translational Psychiatry,* further established BDNF as a key influencer for brain performance. Dr. Salehi, an associate professor of psychiatry and behavioral sciences at Stanford and lead author of the study, noted that while other growth factors and body chemicals were also "up-regulated" by exercise, BDNF seemed to hold the most promise. "The one factor that shows the fastest, most consistent and greatest response is BDNF," he said. "It seems to be key to maintaining not just memory but skilled task performance."[108]

Exercise is unequivocally essential for high performance, so if you are serious about transforming yourself into a high-powered, turbo-charged individual who has high energy and productivity, get on the band wagon of fitness.

Exercise guidelines from the AHA and other groups recommend that you take ten thousand steps or more a day, equivalent to about five miles of walking, to maintain good health. Studies reveal that the majority of adult Americans take fewer than five thousand steps per day.[109]

Not only does exercise improve your mind, enhancing the markers for cognitive abilities like memory, decision making, focus, and attention, it improves your health.

To obtain superior health and a high-functioning brain, exercise regularly. Incorporate it into your daily schedule and protect it with zeal, no matter what obstacles arise. Make it non-negotiable. Don't let your wife, kids, friends, neighbors, coworkers, or clients infringe on it. Get with the program, any program, and start moving!

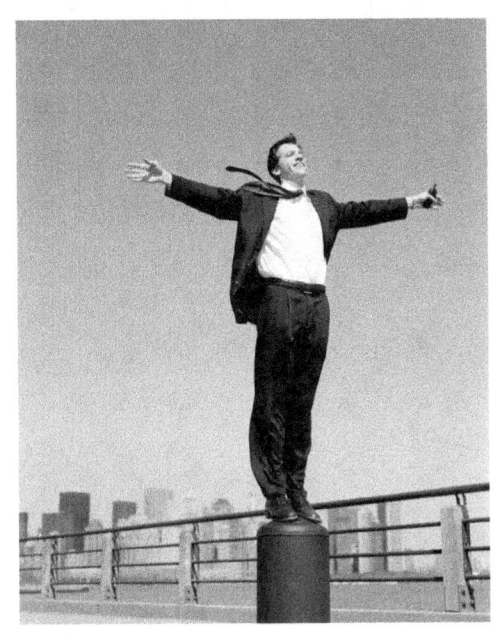

CHAPTER 8:

✧ ✧ ✧

SUPERIOR HEALTH IS BALANCE

STEP 7: MAKE CHOICES THAT MAINTAIN BALANCE.

"Next to love, balance is the most important thing." —*John Wooden*

"Health is sustained by a state of balance among countless strands of a web of genetic, physiological, psychological, developmental, and environmental factors." —**Sidney MacDonald Baker, M.D.**

Superior health is balance. Make conscious choices that help your body, maintain key biological balances, and your brain function, emotional responses, and health will improve dramatically.

CHECKS AND BALANCE

The body and brain are all about balance. The body always seeks to restore homeostasis. *Homeostasis*, meaning "same state," is defined as the tendency of the physiological system to regulate its internal environment and maintain a stable condition, particularly in response to stimulus that might disturb its normal condition.

Our biological systems are constantly in a state of flux. Your body has intricate balancing systems that keep it in check, physiologically speaking, and they work automatically. You never pay attention to how these systems are operating until something is out of balance. Ask people who have type 2 diabetes if they noticed their insulin regulation prior to the onset of their condition. Chances are that they barely noticed how their body regulated blood-sugar levels until it stopped working.

Another example is your thermostat. Your temperature is maintained at 98.6 degrees, in summer and winter. However, if your temperature escalates, as it does on a hot summer day or when you play sports, your body regulates its temperature through your air conditioner, sweat. Sweating brings down your temperature; as the sweat evaporates, it cools the body. Another example is a fever, which is a deliberate escalation of body temperature to exterminate an unwanted virus or bacteria.

In reverse, on a cold winter day, if you do not have the proper insulation, you shiver to increase blood flow and internal temperature. These are the more obvious examples of homeostasis regulation.

When you are in balance, your biological parts work in harmony resulting in high energy, positive emotions and outlook, a strong sense of purpose, and satisfying relationships.

Without balance, you see disturbances in your health and well-being. When something is out of whack, whether emotional or physical, it appears somewhere in your body or brain, and it can put you in distress. If it is emotional, you can have fatigue, headaches, and lack of focus. If it is physiological, you can experience pain, soreness, hives, cold sores, and, in more serious cases, chronic illnesses or disease. Stress alone can create more adverse symptoms than any other state of mind, so coping mechanisms are a critical part of maintaining balance.

Most of the time, you don't have to think about balance because your body does it automatically. However, the world has changed radically in the last sixty years. We live in a world full of chemical toxins; technological, electronic, and information stress; obesity; and dramatic increases in cancer and brain diseases. Even cell phones and computers can cause damage to the brain and/or disrupt sleep patterns because of low levels of radiation or electronic toxicity.

Although balance in all areas—biological, psychological, emotional, spiritual— generate benefits that lead to high performance, in this book we focus on three categories that are critical for your ability to achieve and sustain superior health: energy depletion and renewal, biochemical, and psychological (the latter includes emotional equilibrium, spirituality, and stress management).

1. **Energy expended** during the day is balanced by sleep at night, when the body does **cellular repair work and detoxification.**

2. **Biochemical balance is maintained** with the correct ratio of nutrients, like **omega 3 and omega 6** from fish and olive oil, and a high intake of vegetables, which yield the desired **blood sugar** and **alkaline-to-acid** ratio.

3. **Stress** must be balanced by renewal therapies and **coping skills** (hobbies, exercise, meditation, gardening, sailing, etc.) that restore energy and a positive outlook.

We discussed the first balance of work, energy expenditure, and renewal in previous chapters; that is, the importance of sleep, rest, and relaxing therapies for recharging our energy batteries. We will also address the importance of detoxification for the body and brain in Chapter 9. The remaining two balances are biochemical and psychological.

In the latter category of balance, emotional and spiritual factors both play a significant role in our well-being. However, in the area of physiology, stress is the top interfering element in the quest for achieving balance, so we have isolated *stress management* in this book as one of the important keys to address in HP.

The key biochemical balances are:

1.   Blood Sugar

2.   Acid Alkaline

3.   Omega 3 vs. Omega 6 Fats

A closer look at these balances will give you a better handle on how to influence them. Think about balance as an equation with oppositional forces.

BIOCHEMICAL

1) Blood Sugar Balance   Out of Balance:
Maintains Balance: Refined Sugar,
Complex Carbs +   ⟷   Flour, Rancid Fats,
Good Fats   Excess Protein

2) Alkaline Forming ⟷ Acid Forming
Fruits + Vegetables   Meats, Dairy, Bad Carbs

3) Omega 3 Fats ⟷ Omega 6 Fats
Plants, Nuts, Fish, Seeds   Meats, Poultry, Dairy

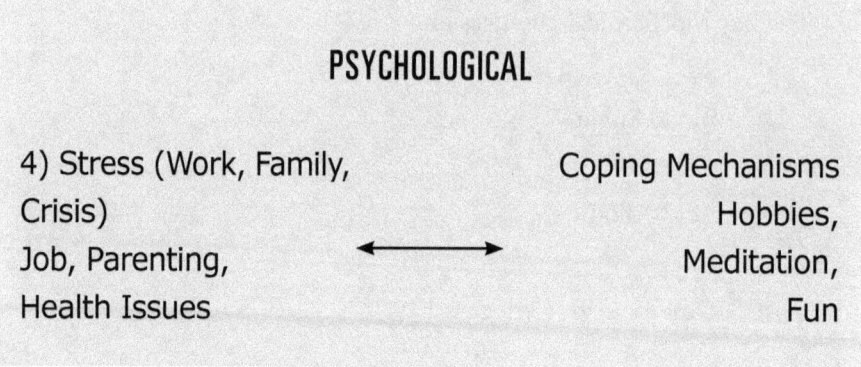

Let's look at each equation separately as a way of defining guide-posts for our health journey.

EQUATION #1: BLOOD SUGAR BALANCE

The importance of blood sugar balance cannot be underestimated; it is one of the keys to superior health, longevity, and high performance.

WHY BLOOD SUGAR BALANCE MATTERS

Blood sugar refers to glucose, and glucose is one of your primary sources of fuel. You know that the brain is a hog (it consumes a disproportionate amount of glucose), so *if you are not providing it with a steady source of high-quality fuel, your brain will not work at its optimal level, and your body may experience dips in energy.*

Blood sugar is also a powerful regulator of immune function, so when your blood sugar balance is disturbed, your ability to fight infection and disease is impacted.[110]

- You have lower levels of white blood cells (associated with a high sugar diet.

- You can have an overgrowth of yeast and bacteria when you eat too many starches and sweets, because carbohydrates are the preferred food of many microbes.

- Your susceptibility to cancer increases, because cancer cells feed on sugar.[111]

- You damage your immune function because of the internal chain reactions that involve overproduction of insulin and other hormones. Besides stressing your metabolic systems, these reactions can also inhibit antibody production, which is your defense team for fighting invaders like viruses and bacteria.

Major research confirms that diet and poor blood sugar regulation are important risk factors for adult-onset type 2 diabetes.[112] This condition is prevalent in Western populations and on the rise.

Blood sugar imbalances occur when you eat excessive amounts of bad carbs (simple carbohydrates). Your white enemy is the foods that are processed heavily to maintain shelf life, devoid of nutrients, full of trans fats, and have a high content of white, refined sugar, and simple starches. The result? Our modern diet (also called the SAD diet, no pun intended, for Standard American Diet) wreaks havoc with blood sugar balance, giving many people blood sugar highs and lows every day.

ANOTHER WORD ABOUT SUGAR "CRACK": THE SHORT-LIVED ENERGY RUSH DEPLETES INSULIN

When blood sugar (glucose) is too high, the body is forced to bring it down, so it releases excessive amounts of insulin, a hormone produced by the pancreas. The price is high. The body must dispose of the hormone, so some of the blood sugar is expended as energy, but most of it, because it is not quality energy and usually in excess of what your body needs, is converted and stored as fat, the arch nemesis of good health and fitness.

Research shows that this process is one of the primary causes of weight gain. More importantly, it is also a form of metabolic stress that creates unwanted toxins.

Let's look at the flip side of this coin. The stability of blood sugar has positive effects on important HP markers:

Mood
Mental clarity
Energy
Allergic sensitivities
Metabolism
Weight management
Heart health

Maintaining blood sugar balance is not difficult if you follow the prescription for superior health:

- Eat good carbs; they give you quality energy.
- Avoid bad carbs; they rob you of energy and hook you on sugar.
- Have a regular eating schedule, and eat high-quality snacks.
- Eat quality foods that provide both macrofuel *and* microfuel.
- Exercise; it helps regulate blood sugar balance.

EQUATION #2: ACID-ALKALINE BALANCE

We have all heard about the pH in our shampoos but there is also a pH in our bodies, which is the state of equilibrium maintained in our body fluids in order to carry out vital cellular activities. This balance is required because most of the metabolic processes produce acids as their end products, and these acids must be neutralized, exchanged or eliminated.

Just as our body maintains a certain temperature, our blood has an optimal pH (defined in biological terms as hydrogen ion concentration) between 7.35 and 7.45. If we fail to achieve this balance, the enzyme systems and our other biochemical and metabolic activities will not function correctly or optimally.

The importance of the acid alkaline balance to your health can be summed up in this statement: The more acidic you are, that is, the more **acidic wastes** you accumulate, the more susceptible you are to degenerative diseases and chronic illness. The more alkaline you are, the better your overall health, and the longer your ability to live a healthy life.

This fact is supported by an experiment conducted by a Nobel Prize-winning surgeon and biologist, **Alexis Carrell**.[113] The experiment, conducted with pieces of a chicken heart tissue, is cited by many scientists as demonstrating the "immortality" of the cell, because the tissue was kept alive for twenty-eight years.

Carrell kept pieces of heart tissue alive in a solution containing the same mineral levels found in chicken blood plasma, changing the solution daily to eliminate acidic wastes. Carrell claimed that the heart cells could not sustain life with just nutrients and the correct minerals alone, because the metabolic activities of the heart would produce acidic wastes that would pollute the fluid in which they were placed. By changing this fluid, and removing the acidic wastes, the heart cells flourished for twenty-eight years. The cells died when an assistant forgot to change the fluid and remove the wastes.

THE SIGNIFICANCE OF THE CARRELL EXPERIMENT

Human organs are surrounded by fluids that deliver nutrients to the cells while simultaneously removing metabolic wastes, like the chicken heart experiment. The theory Carrell postulated, and as espoused by many scientists, is that human cells need both the correct amount of nutrients and a clean fluid (extracellular) environment. The accumulation of acidic wastes pollutes the fluids of the body, resulting in the demise of cells, tissues, and organs.

The experiment demonstrated the important relationship between metabolic wastes and nutrition. No matter how well you are nourished, if your body produces wastes that are not removed (detoxification), the cells degenerate and die.

Let's look at it another way.

Although both acid and alkaline substances are vital to life, acidity favors the decomposition of living things, while alkali prevents it. In her book, *The Acid Alkaline Balance Diet,* Felicia Kliment cites the state of corpses found buried in the fourteenth century under the Cathedral of Venzone in Italy as an example of the importance of alkalinity. While some of the corpses remained intact, others became skeletons. The puzzle was easily solved. "The dead bodies interred when the underground water contained a high concentration of alkaline-forming lime became mummified, whereas the flesh of the bodies buried in places where the water is highly acidic was eaten away by bacteria." Kliment found "the common denominator in all degenerative diseases: acidic wastes." [114]

You want your body to maintain a higher alkalinity on balance, which favors cell maintenance and renewal. You also want to avoid creating an internal environment that is acidic.

Pretty simple formula. Now you just have to learn what produces acidic wastes in the body, what produces alkalinity, and how to control both to the degree that you can with your conscious choices.

ALKALINITY: YOUR ALLY IN SUPERIOR HEALTH

We have established that what you ingest and manufacture in terms of toxins produces acids and alkaline, so the next question to ask is: how can you control this balance?

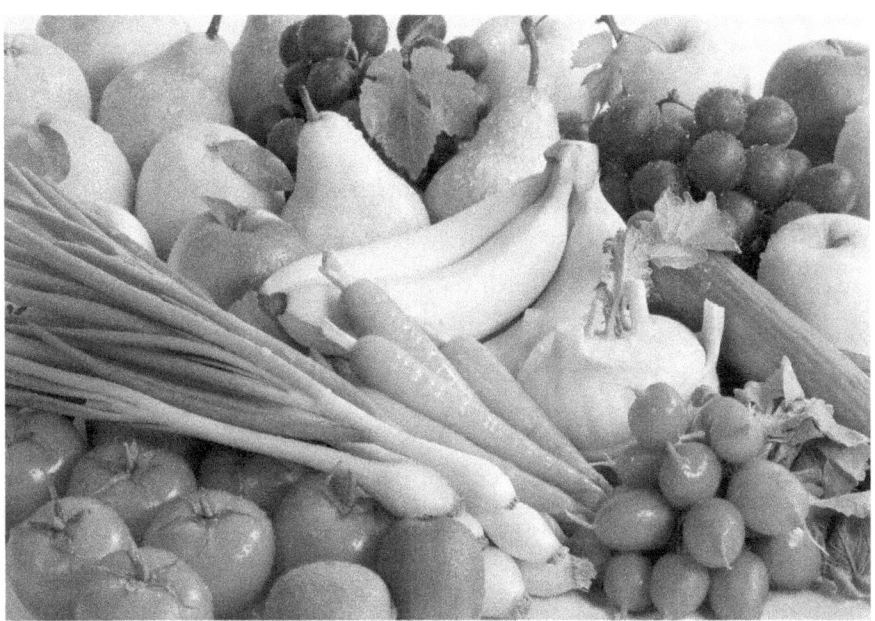

The easiest answer, and the one you have heard before, is that you should eat lots of fruits and vegetables. Why? *Because—fruits and vegetables are alkalizing!*

Think of the corpses mentioned by Kliment. When interred in lime, an alkaline environment, the corpses showed little decomposition. When in an acidic environment, the corpses deteriorated and were eaten by bacteria.

This is a grisly picture, but that is exactly what you should think of when you are eating. More alkaline is produced with a diet high in vegetables. The more alkaline you are, the healthier you are. All your cells and organs are surrounded by fluids and contain fluids. These fluids can be in balance (more alkaline to acid) or out of balance (more acid to alkaline). Which would you prefer?

What can you do to reduce and eliminate acid production? Seek and destroy the "white enemies" in your refrigerator, cupboard, and plate. They usually come in a package filled with preservatives and food coloring; they are definitely acid forming. Protein is also acid forming, but you need protein, and what's important is to keep your protein intake in alignment with your vegetable/fruit intake.

If you are eating a hamburger, French fries, with a cola, these are all acid-forming foods. Where is your balance? Where is your raw green salad? If you do have a salad, does it represent 10 percent of your food intake or 50 percent? If you want to maintain a good ratio between acid and alkaline, the meat, French fries, and cola should be the smallest percentage of your meal, not 75–80 percent. The opposite is also true. If you want to maintain an alkaline balance, remember the color principle and the "one ingredient" rule: the more color on your plate, the more single ingredients in your refrigerator, the more alkaline you become, the healthier you are, and the more energy you have. You should always strive to keep your body slightly alkaline in order to build an alkaline reserve for acid-forming conditions, such as stress, lack of exercise, or poor dietary habits.

ACID VERSUS ALKALINE FOODS

If you get into this subject, you will find some differences of opinion among scientists and cultures regarding which foods are acid forming and which are alkaline forming. Our view is that you need to learn which foods are helpful in reducing acidic wastes, regardless of whether they are acid or alkaline producing. We want to spotlight the fact that you accumulate acidic wastes from low-quality foods, toxins, and free radicals.

Your job is to learn about these by-products and make choices that enable your body to maintain a higher alkalinity ratio.

An example of the differences of opinion surfaces when you look at how the body metabolizes certain vegetables. As we pointed out, the most alkaline-producing foods are fruits and vegetables, with emphasis on sprouts, cereal grasses, and herbs. However, the juice of carrots and beets, although they have a high percentage of acid-forming sulphur and phosphorus, effectively clean out the acidic wastes from the liver, kidneys, and bladder. Similarly, the juice of cabbage, although high in acidic chlorine and sulphur, cleanses the acid wastes adhering to the mucous membranes of the stomach and intestinal tract. Other effective cleansers include alkaline minerals, like potassium, calcium, sodium and magnesium. These minerals are found in dandelions, endive, and lettuce; they all reduce the hyperacidity in all the organs of the body.[115,116] (Think about an ordinary household cleaner made of bicarbonate of soda (alkaline) and vinegar(acid). They act together to clean.

EQUATION #3: OMEGA 3 TO OMEGA-6 FATS

WHY IT'S SUCH A BALANCING ACT

These are your "smart fats," because your brain uses them for firing messages and all kinds of processes associated with HP. They are the essential fats you need for your operating systems, and they cannot be manufactured in your body.

OMEGA 3: SMART FATS CRITICAL FOR HIGH PERFORMANCE

Let's review briefly why omega 3 fats are so important. They compose the myelin sheath, which are important to brain cells (remember, the brain does a lot of signalling). However, omega 3 is not only part of the insulation in your brain wiring, it is also the raw material for prostaglandins, those powerful hormone regulators we mentioned earlier.

Prostaglandins are known to relax blood vessels (which lowers blood pressure, **particularly important if you want to manage stress**), and they help you maintain water balance. They also **boost immunity,** they **decrease inflammation and pain** (for those with arthritis or back problems), and **they help balance blood sugar** by improving insulin effectiveness. Prostaglandins also regulate the release and **performance of neurotransmitters,** and low levels are known to be involved in conditions including depression.

There are three types of these fatty acids: ALA, EPA, and DHA. Omega 3 is the patriarch of the omega family, and it is the alpha-linolenic acid (ALA) fatty acid that produces the metabolically active offspring of eicosapentenoic acid (EPA) and docasahexenoic acid (DHA). They can be differentiated by the number of carbons in each chain:

ALA-ALA: 18-carbon chain

EPA-EPA: 20-carbon chain

DHA-DHA: 22-carbon chain

Well, you will never need to remember the carbon chain, or even these long names, but you should remember what each of these 3 types of omega-3's does for your health:

The **ALA** omega-3 helps **reduce heart disease and stroke** by reducing cholesterol and triglyceride levels, enhancing the elasticity of blood vessels, and preventing the build-up of harmful fat deposits in the arteries.

EPA and **DHA** help with **brain and eye development, prevent cardiovascular disease, and help prevent Alzheimer's disease.** Research shows that diets high in DHA protect against degenerative processes within the retina.

Other studies showed that populations with higher intake of DHA/EPA experienced an approximate 40 percent reduction in cardiovascular disease and a significant reduction in all-cause mortality.

Omega 3 fatty acids can also correct imbalances in modern diets that lead to heart disease, stroke, and cancer. Omega 3 fats, according to brain specialists, affect learning, behavior, attention deficit disorder, and schizophrenia. They also help lower LDL, the "bad" cholesterol.

What is the importance of these fats to the brain and high performance?

ONE-QUARTER OF THE WEIGHT OF THE BRAIN IS DHA.

ALA is found in oils of flax, pumpkin, and walnuts. Its offspring, EPA and DHA, are found in fish and fish oils. The primary sources of EPA and DHA are cold-water fish, especially fish that eat fish (which is why seals, which eat small fish, are so rich in EPA and DHA, and why the Inuit population in Alaska has the lowest risk of heart disease).

According to Holford, the best diet for a high-functioning brain is a "fishatarian" (pescetarian) or a high seed (particularly flaxseed) diet so that you can obtain the necessary levels of omega 3 fats.[117] In the twenty-first century, we eat excessive amounts of processed fats, packaged meats, and foods devoid of this nutrient, which is the root of our balancing problems.

OMEGA 6 VERSUS OMEGA 3

Omega 6 is the other essential fatty acid you must obtain from the food you eat. Like omega 3, it is a polyunsaturated fat, but unlike 3, it is more readily available. You can obtain it directly from eating meat, poultry, and eggs, as well as nut and plant-based oils such as canola and sunflower.

Of all the tissues in the body, the brain has the highest percentage of this fat. The important fact about omega 6 fat is that too much of it causes inflammation, and inflammation is damaging to the body and brain.[118, 119,120]

Today, people over consume foods with a high percentage of omega 6, and they don't even begin to get enough omega 3.

What is wrong with this picture? You have one fat in excess, and one fat in deficient amounts. You usually have an excess of omega 6 and a distressingly low level of the brain-boosting, immune-enhancing omega 3.

According to the NIH, the US diet no longer contains the amount of omega 3 fatty acids that the body needs for overall health and wellness. The average person eats one-sixth the omega 3 fats found in the diet of people living in 1850.

Instead of a balanced ratio of 3 to 6 (which promotes lower risk of chronic disease, prevents heart disease, stroke, and cancer), you have higher amounts of omega 6, a known factor in promoting heart disease, high cholesterol, depression, asthma, arthritis, and Alzheimer's disease.[121]

WHY OMEGA 3 IS DEFICIENT IN MODERN DIETS

Here comes the reality check and a point which bears repeating: the average person today eats one-sixth the omega 3 fats found in the diet of people living in 1850.

There are three reasons for this:

1. The modern diet has seen a dramatic increase in meat and a decrease in fresh produce. Meats are abundant in omega 6, so you usually get an ample supply of this omega. In contrast, omega 3s come from plants, nuts, and fish. The average person consumes

one or two servings of vegetables and fruits a day instead of the recommended five to six servings.

- We have changed from a vegetable, rice, and grain diet to a more meat-centric, packaged-food diet. This too has resulted in drastic reductions in omega 3.

2. The animals you are eating are not grazing on grass (rich in omega 3s) but are fed soy and corn (omega 6), laced with antibiotics. Since the Industrial Age, farming practices switched from grass-fed, small farms to large scale, commercial operations using soy and corn feed (cheaper) for beef, veal, pork, and other meats. Dairy is no longer a source of omega 3s. If you lived in your grandmother's day, you would also get omega 3s from chickens, eggs, butter, and milk. For the chickens and cows, grass supplied a rich abundance of omega 3s and other vital minerals, whereas corn and soy provide omega 6s.

3. Cooking, heating, and food processing can damage the more delicate omega 3 fats, because they are more unsaturated and therefore more prone to damage.

- These factors have led to an imbalance between the 3s and 6s, causing a deleterious impact on health.

And just to get that broken record effect again, the reason why the balancing act between the 3's and 6's is so important is *because too much omega 6 fatty acid can contribute to inflammation and result in heart disease, cancer, asthma, arthritis, and depression.*

So what can we do?

Become more aware of your food sources and the quality of your nutrients. In the quest for high performance, it is no longer about the calories but the quality of the nutrients, particularly the micronutrients, that are responsible for fine-tuning your body's functions and the quality of your brain patterns.

If you are designing an omega 3-rich, brain-boosting food program, incorporate cold-water fish like salmon, mackerel, herring, sardines, anchovies, and tuna (the Japanese have three times the omega 3 fats in their body fat compared to the average American), as well as seeds from linseed (flax), hemp, and pumpkin. Walnuts are also a rich source of omega 3.

Be aware that although both omega 3 and omega 6 fats are essential, the omega 3 fat is harder to come by. Actively find ways to increase your consumption of foods with high levels of omega 3, or take supplements, to maintain adequate amounts in your diet.

EQUATION #4: STRESS VERSUS RENEWAL THERAPIES AND COPING SKILLS

The complex relationship between physical and psychological health is not well understood. Scientists know that psychological stress can affect the immune system and lower defenses against infection and diseases like cancer.

There are several types of stress, and not all of them are harmful, because sometimes the adrenaline from stress can protect you or instigate creativity. We define stress as any type of change or experience that causes one of four types of strain:

1) Physical (exertion doing a physical activity)

2) Emotional (death, divorce, moving, etc.)

3) Psychological (work, management, financial crisis, etc.)

4)   Physiological (toxins, disease, chronic inflammation, etc.)

Positive stress is called *eustress*. It is the type of stress that you encounter when doing something fun and exciting, anything from riding a roller coaster or skiing down a challenging slope to doing an interview on television or meeting a deadline. You need this kind of stress in your life; it is exciting and keeps you vital.

There are three other types of stress that can have a negative effect on your health:[122]

Acute. This is the short-term kind of stress that you encounter in everyday life like having a flat tire, traffic, being called into a meeting unexpectedly without preparation, or presenting a business proposal to a hostile board of directors.

Episodic. This is continuous, acute stress, where life is constantly filled with aggravating or situational problems that yield perpetual anxiety. There is probably someone in your life whose day-to-day pattern resembles this; he or she usually falls into the category of "drama queen" or "stress case."

Chronic stress. This is the type of stress that you encounter most often in high-level executives, business owners, and anyone with a demanding career. It is usually pervasive in the person's life. It might be caused by a high-profile job with continuous demands. It can also be from a bad relationship or financial pressures that seem inescapable. This type of stress can cause severe health problems and lead to "burn-out"—characterized by adrenal exhaustion; insomnia; depression; and chronic back-aches, headaches, etc.

WHAT STRESS DOES TO YOUR BODY AND BRAIN

The body responds to stress by releasing stress hormones like epinephrine (adrenaline) and cortisol (hydrocortisone). You produce these stress hormones to react to a harmful situation with more speed and strength. In doing so, the hormones increase blood pressure, heart rate, and blood sugar levels. They slow digestion and redirect blood flow to major muscle groups, allowing you to flee a predator or confront impending danger.

Stress is an autonomic nervous response; that is, you do not control it because it is programmed into your DNA (hardwired) to give us this burst of energy and strength in order to flee a predator or confront impending danger. The "fight or flight" response is the body's trigger to perceived danger.

Although this automatic response is intended to protect you, it is now activated on a more routine basis. In a crazy, technologically and stress-filled world, response mechanisms are often triggered by real stress (crime in big cities) or perceived stress—traffic while commuting, being late for an important meeting, demands on the job, deadlines, etc. If the "fight or flight" response is triggered continuously, even when it is not appropriate, the threat is no longer an external one; it now endangers your internal environment and your health.

More importantly, chronic stress disables your ability to readjust your settings and relax. When the perceived threat is gone, your homeostasis mechanisms (the ones that keep everything in balance, designed to trigger the relaxation response) become disabled. The relaxation response is muted or does not kick in. The body keeps responding to stress by releasing stress hormones, but the counter-responses are not working. (Think of what happens when you are in the middle of typing a Word document, and your computer freezes, alerting you by signalling "Not Responding.")

Although small amounts of stress are believed to be beneficial, chronic stress that gets worse over time take its toll on the body.[123]

According to Elizabeth Scott, author of 8 Keys to Stress Management, when you are faced with chronic stress, you overstimulate the "fight or flight" response, triggering stress hormones too frequently, resulting in stress-influenced conditions that include the following:[124]

- Depression
- Diabetes
- Hair loss
- Heart disease
- Hyperthyroidism
- Obesity
- Obsessive-compulsive or anxiety disorder
- Sexual dysfunction
- Tooth and gum disease
- Ulcers
- Cancer

Chronic stress can start with simple symptoms that are easily ignored: frequent headaches, stomach issues, and lowered immunity (causing more colds and other sicknesses). Over time, these symptoms escalate and interfere with the quality of your everyday life.[125]

STRESS MANAGEMENT AND COPING MECHANISMS

Strategy 1

The first step in managing stress is to get a handle on how you react to it. Put the proverbial mirror up to your behavior, and observe yourself in stressful situations as though you were detached from your body. Do you shout and get angry? Do you panic? Do you curse like a sailor and look for something to kick? Do you move away from confrontation and internalize your anger?

Some people take everything in stride, others internalize, and others externalize. Take an honest look at yourself and your stress management style. Does it serve you, or do you need to modify your technique so that stress doesn't lead to serious health issues?

Here are some common but unhealthy reactions to stress.

Pain. You develop unexplained physical pain or a number of other health problems. Common conditions include upset stomach, painful knots in the abdomen, shortness of breath, muscle tension, especially in the neck and upper shoulder area, back pain, headaches, and insomnia. Sound familiar?

Over/under eating. Stress can trigger habitual eating, even when you are not hungry, or the opposite—you may eat less and lose weight.

Anger. If you have a short fuse, this is another indication of chronic stress. When pressure intensifies, you may discover that you argue with everyone in your orbit, including coworkers, friends, and family members, even though the things you argue about are not related to the stressful situation.

Depression. Sometimes stress can make you feel that your problems are hopeless, and you feel overwhelmed, which can lead to depression and anxiety disorders.

Crying. Stress can provoke spontaneous and uncontrollable crying episodes. Small things can trigger an episode and result in feelings of isolation and exasperation.

Negative outlook. Chronic stress can impact mood. Producing more stress hormones wreaks havoc with your mood regulators and your serotonin levels (the "calm-me-down" hormone). You may start to have ANTs in all situations, anticipating the worst outcome for everything.

Smoking and drinking. These are often linked to stress. A cigarette or a stiff drink may seem like a socially acceptable way to relax and ease the pressure. On closer inspection, smoking and drinking are temporary fixes and usually "turn up the volume." You do not do anything constructive to resolve the stress, and you have not implemented an effective coping mechanism to manage your state of mind.[126]

Stress usually doesn't magically get better on its own. Pills, liquor, and recreational drugs are not healthy ways to cope; they lead you farther from your HP goals, because they damage your brain. Decide to actively work on getting control of the stress in your life, or it will control you. Once you identify how you react to stressful situations and become more aware of your behavior, you will be in a better position to manage the stress, if you can't eliminate it. If your efforts at stress management aren't working, try something new.

Strategy 2

If you are satisfied with your coping skills, skip this part. If you are not sure, keep a journal for a week or so and observe your reactions to stressful situations. It's important to know how you react to stress first before you can improve your skills. If you want to learn new skills or modify your behavior, keep reading.

There are lots of stress management techniques. The trick, as with changing your fuel portfolio, is to identify, assess, experiment, and decide. Identify what techniques are available, assess which ones might work, experiment with different ones to determine their effectiveness for you, and decide to integrate them into your skill set for living life more abundantly.

Here are some actions you can take to manage stress in the short term.

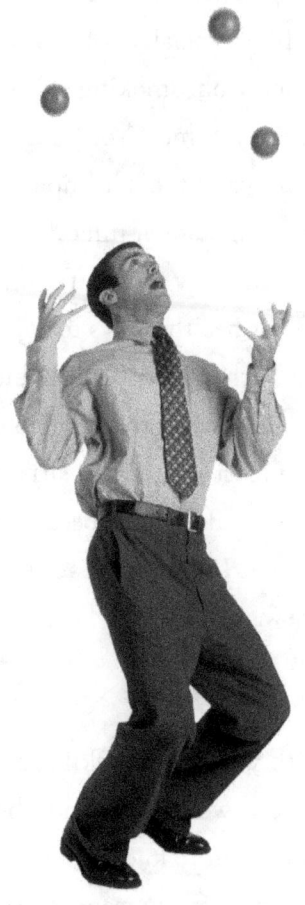

- **Prioritize your crystal balls and rubber balls.** Make a list of
  the important obligations and projects in your life: family, mar-
  riage, kids and their associated activities, job, management responsibilities, etc. Then make a list of important things that take
  a lot of your time and focus. Look at the lists and decide which
  obligations, if push came to shove, could be dropped or resched-
  uled, without damage, and which are too important to tamper
  with and could be harmed if ignored or "dropped."

Divide the list into "crystal balls" and "rubber balls." The crystal balls are the important obligations that cannot be dropped because they are crystal—too precious and delicate—and might break. The rest can bounce, because they are rubber balls—the obligations that recover. Now you have a strategy for determining where you put your focus and energy when you are stressed about conflicts in your life. You can use this strategy as a general rule or on a case-by-case basis.

- **Scale back.** Scrutinize your daily, weekly, and monthly schedule, and identify the meetings, dinner obligations, functions, and chores that can be delegated or pared back to give you more time and flexibility. This task is especially difficult for high performers because they like to be in control, multitasking their schedules to the nth degree. As you scale back, your quality of life and usually the quality of your work improve. Pay attention to energy drains, and cut back on obligations wherever possible.

- **Anticipate and prepare.** Jump ahead of your schedule and deadlines as often as possible. If you can anticipate delays or time crunches, you improve your schedule and avoid stressful circumstances. This means preparing in advance for meetings, trips, speeches, and papers, and it means scheduling your time better. Leave extra time for arriving at airports and important meetings. Set realistic goals and timelines for tasks big and small. Stress often rears its ugly head when you run out of time because something comes up that you didn't account for, so build in time for traffic jams, or management jams.

- **Galvanize your support network.** The importance of a network of supportive family, friends, and colleagues cannot be underestimated in its ability to support you. Renew and maintain positive connections with others. Surround yourself with people who have a positive effect on your well-being and ability to cope with stress.

- **Relax, work, relax: It's all about balance.** Relaxation is an essential part of high-performance balance. Physical activity, meditation, yoga, massage, fishing, skinny dipping, skydiving, or any relaxation technique that works for you can help manage stress. Cast your net for relaxation devices as far and wide as suits you; it doesn't matter which techniques you choose. What matters is that the techniques allow you to refocus on something that keeps you calm or distracted and relaxes you.

- **Take up a new hobby or rediscover an old hobby.** This dovetails with relaxing techniques, because a hobby engages your mind, and usually your hands, in doing something soothing. It is a great strategy for managing stress. It can be as simple as playing with a miniature basketball hoop in your office or painting. It can be tinkering with electronics, fishing, carpentry, knitting, or listening to music. When you engage in something enjoyable, it can soothe your restless mind. It may sound cliché, but the things that you do for fun are one of the best ways to deal with stress.

- **Learn new, tension-relief techniques.** You will discover that there are many techniques to activate your relaxation response. Meditation, yoga, deep breathing, journaling, and invoking positive imagery are at the top of the list. These are proven techniques that help you feel more relaxed; it's just a matter of finding which ones suit your temperament.

- **Get sleep for your sanity and well-being.** Lack of sufficient sleep affects your immune system and judgment. It also affects your mood and ability to cope with everyday situations. You may erupt like a volcano over minor irritations. Most people need seven to eight hours of sleep each night.

- **Learn good organization, time-management, and relationship-building skills.** Although some acute stress is unavoidable and less predictable, episodic and chronic stress, the kinds that damage health, can be avoided or minimized once you sharpen some your skills for day-to-day situations. For example, learn how to be more persuasive so that your effectiveness goes up. Manage your time by becoming better organized and focused and avoid time-wasting events; your efficiency will increase. Once your organization and relationship skills improve, your stress will decrease proportionately.

- **Seek professional help.** If you have tried and failed to apply stress-management techniques, seek a professional who can help you. Chronic stress, like any chronic health problem, can lead to serious health issues such as depression and pain.

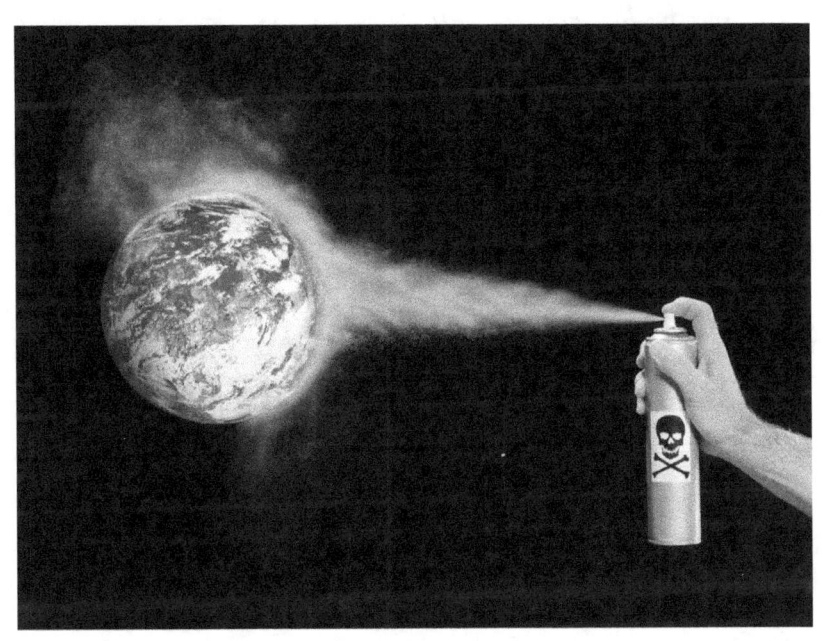

CHAPTER 9:

✯ ✯ ✯

DETOXIFICATION

STEP 8: BEWARE OF TOXINS, AND USE METHODS TO ASSIST NATURAL DETOXIFICATION.

"Balance means providing all the necessary elements to optimize the system and remove any interfering elements. Nutrients are necessary elements. Toxins are interfering elements."

"Of all the functions in human biology there is one overriding function that connects to all the others. Understanding its chemistry and immunology can unify the physician's approach to problems of any level of complexity. It is detoxification." [127] —Sidney McDonald Baker, MD

"We are living in a sea of toxins, and there is good evidence that this is affecting our health in a major way. Many chronic conditions such as arthritis, <u>chronic fatigue</u>, fibromyalgia, elevated cholesterol and triglycerides, <u>depression</u> and on and on are related to our toxic world. These chemical toxins are stored in fat in the body and are likely a major contributing factor to the obesity epidemic in the US and the world." [128] —Dr. Marsha Nunley

"The two most important things you need to know to cure disease, create health, and lose weight are:
1. *The role of <u>nutrition</u> in health and disease.*
2. *The role of toxins and <u>the importance of detoxification</u> in health and disease."*

"Unfortunately, you probably aren't going to learn much about them from your doctor. Most physicians today are still hopelessly ignorant in these areas. They were simply never taught about nutrition and detoxification in medical school." —Mark Hyman, MD[129]

"We believe in first trying to determine possible triggers for health issues and patterns of behavior that lead to illness. Oftentimes this will lead to an assisted Detoxification intervention strategy in order to eliminate what might be disturbing the body's system. Detoxification, if done correctly, can "reboot" the body's biochemistry, re-establish balance, and restart the body's metabolic machinery, so to speak." —Jill Karlsson Kazikos, holistic nutrition and functional medicine therapist

DETOXIFICATION 101

Detoxification is essential for high performance.

We discussed the importance of repair and detoxification during sleep. We also discussed the balance of what goes in (nutrition and toxins) and what goes out (detoxification, elimination).

Everyone is equipped with detoxification machinery, and you would not be able to survive without it. You are exposed to hundreds of toxins every day. Internally, they occur as the by-product of foods, the break-down and/or repair of cells, and from emotions like stress, sadness, and depression. Externally, they come from toxic chemicals in the air you breathe, the clothes you wear, viruses, bacteria, pesticides, antibiotics, heavy metals, and anything else that gets into your body and interferes with balance.

DETOXIFICATION: SANITATION AND ENEMY REMOVAL SYSTEM

Detoxification is the "saw" in the "see saw." You eat, breathe, move, grow, wear out cells, and repair them; you are always creating metabolic waste, and you are always exposed to environmental toxins. Research reveals that you replace a million cells a day!

The balance between what goes in (see) and what goes out (saw) is handled by the body's natural detoxification machinery. If this process works properly, and all that is harmful is removed promptly and efficiently, the body's internal machinery works like a Swiss clock: very efficiently.

When the machinery is not working, or when it is overburdened due to toxic overload, you experience problems that can manifest as illness, disease, allergies or a chronic condition like rheumatoid arthritis.

Detoxification is the biggest item in the biochemical budget. The body is constantly removing wastes from the environment and from every process in the organs and systems. Almost every molecule the body deals with has to be removed when it has served its purpose.

When your digestive system breaks down a protein into amino acids, the waste product is ammonia. Because ammonia is *not* something you want lingering in your body, your detoxification machinery renders the molecule inactive and pushes it out. When your hormones are no longer needed by the endocrine system, they become garbage and must be removed.

What happens to the germs you are exposed to every day? What about the virus that you caught that ended up as a running nose? The running nose is the end of the body's detoxification work: your immune system has "tagged and bagged" those nasty bugs, and its way of removing them is to neutralize and recycle them as waste product that is pushed out with mucous—hence, the running nose.

Detoxification is particularly vital to the functioning of your immune system. When it works, your health is strong. When it is compromised, you can get sick.

One of the main processes of your body is troubleshooting for toxins that look like innocent molecules but are instead dangerous trespassers that have escaped detection. Your immune system depends on the ability of your "seek and destroy" immune cells to identify and isolate viral and bacterial invaders. It depends on the detoxification process to neutralize and remove the toxic wastes.

A state of balance is maintained when all your detoxification systems are working optimally; this is why detoxification is one of the most important functions in your body and why it is the most costly, in terms of metabolic activity. It requires the lion's share of energy to make the molecules to remove waste products and molecular invaders.

Ordinarily, your detoxification machinery (which resides mainly in the liver, kidneys, lungs, small intestine, skin, lymph system, and intestinal lining) can destroy or debilitate unwanted substances. However, if your detoxification equipment is overloaded or not functioning correctly, you have a problem: the toxins, also described here as "the interfering elements," cannot be properly or expediently removed, so they wreak havoc with your internal balance and operating systems for health.

Think back to the Carrell experiment we talked about in Chapter 8. The most important insight gained after 28 years of research on the chicken heart was this: if the correct supply of nutrients is provided, the heart can be maintained indefinitely. However, if the metabolic wastes are not removed daily, the fluids surrounding the cells create an acidic environment, which is not conducive with sustaining the metabolic activities of life. *The heart died after 28 years only when acidic wastes were not removed.*

THE PROBLEM OF TOXINS IN THE TWENTY-FIRST CENTURY

We are exposed to chemicals every day. They are in the food you eat, the air you breathe, the water you drink, and the lotions you put on your skin. They can coat the surface of dust particles, so you can inhale them when you breathe (particularly if you live in cities where the exhaust from buses and cars causes pollution). They can be in products like cosmetics, clothes dry-cleaned with solvents, plastic food containers, home and garden pesticides, and paints and varnishes.

There are four categories of toxins:

1) Toxins from food fuel (everything from ammonia with protein metabolism to hormones given to the animals you eat, pesticide residue, and food coloring)

2) Toxins from cellular repair

3) Toxins from the external environment (shampoos, dry cleaning solvents, pharmaceuticals, air pollution, and molecular invaders)

4) Toxins from emotions (anger, sadness, stress, trauma)

TOXINS: THE INTERFERING ELEMENTS

We know that toxins come from our food because they are burned and absorbed (metabolized). Every food molecule creates waste by-products. Some of these wastes are toxic and must be neutralized, and some are removed like trash and expunged from the body. The toxins are unavoidable, and your detoxification machinery is prepared to safely dispose of them.

However, a seemingly harmless new category of food substances has also become toxic: the "new" food chemicals that the body does not recognize or cannot digest properly. These include high fructose corn syrup, trans fats, food coloring, monosodium glutamate (MSG), aspartame and artificial sweeteners, and preservatives.[130,131]

All of these food chemicals interfere with the body's metabolism and can create a multitude of problems unless removed by the body's detoxification machinery.

TOXINS FROM THE ENVIRONMENT

Toxins from the environment can be anything from a grain of pollen, which your body removes with sneezing, or chemicals that are in your foods, on your clothes, or in the air.

Below is a list of findings that illuminate the problem of toxins in our environment and underscore the concurrent and implicit necessity for detoxification and cleansing. These facts are reported by the EPA, the Environmental Working Group (EWG), National Resources Defense Council (NRDC), the US government, and REACH, the European Community regulation on chemicals (Registration, Evaluation, Authorisation and Restriction of Chemical substances).[132,133]

1. The Environmental Protection Agency's (EPA's) Toxic Substance Control Act (TSCA) Chemical Substances Inventory lists information on more than sixty-two thousand chemicals or chemical substances; some libraries maintain files of material safety data sheets (MSDS) for more than one hundred thousand substances. OSHA currently regulates exposure to approximately *four hundred substances*[134]
    United States Department of Labor

2. "The US produces or imports close to three thousand chemicals (excluding polymers and inorganic chemicals) at over one

million pounds per year. EPA's analysis found that no basic toxicity information, i.e., neither human health nor environmental toxicity, is publicly available for 43 percent of the high-volume chemicals manufactured in the US and that *a full set of basic toxicity information is available for only 7 percent of these chemicals.*" [135]

Chemical Hazard Data Availability Study

3. "Chemicals have always been regulated due to the strong potential link between chemicals and a wide range of diseases, including respiratory and bladder cancers, eye and skin disorders, and asthma. Existing chemicals (approximately 100,000 reported) required no testing before marketing. Only new chemicals were tested in a rigorous manner. As a result, little is known about the hazards of existing chemicals."[136]

Registration, Evaluation, and Authorization of Chemicals (REACH)

4. "Quite a few cleaning products that line store shelves are packed with toxic chemicals that can wreak havoc with your health, including many that harm the lungs." [137]

Environmental Working Group senior scientist Rebecca Sutton

5. EWG found that slightly more than half of the cleaning products they tested contained ingredients known to be harmful to lungs. Products that contain chlorine bleach can sometimes release chloroform, which is thought to be a human carcinogen. [138]

Environmental Working Group 2012 Guide to Healthy Cleaning

6. "It seems clear that hazardous pollutants contribute to the large and growing toll of chronic conditions, such as cancers and heart disease. Chemical pollutants can also play a role in infectious diseases, perhaps by rendering the body less able to ward off infections."[139]
National Resources Defense Council

7. When combined, chemicals are even more dangerous. Deadly fumes result from mixing ammonia with bleach (both found in many household products) creating lethal "mustard gas"![140]
US Government, EPA

8. Petrochemical cleaning products in the home are easily absorbed into the skin. Once absorbed, the toxins travel to the blood stream and are deposited in the fatty tissues where they may exist indefinitely.[141]

9. The American Cancer Society reports that environmental factors can account for three-quarters of all cancers.[142]

10. Scientists estimate that everyone alive today carries within her or his body at least seven hundred contaminants, most of which have not been well studied.[143]

11. Research conducted by the Environmental Working Group and reported by Joseph Mercola found 232 toxins in newborns: "In all, the tests found as many as 232 chemicals in the ten

newborns, all of minority descent. The cord blood study has produced hard new evidence that American children are being exposed, beginning in the womb, to complex mixtures of dangerous substances that may have lifelong consequences."[144]

12. Some chemicals or their breakdown products (metabolites) lodge in the body for only a short while before being excreted, but continuous exposure to such chemicals can create a "persistent" body burden. Arsenic, for example, is mostly excreted within seventy-two hours of exposure. However, other chemicals are not readily excreted and can remain for years in your blood, adipose (fat) tissue, semen, muscle, bone, brain tissue, or other organs. The term "body burden" refers to the total amount of these chemicals present in the human body at a given point in time.[145]

13. The average home contains sixty-two toxic chemicals, more than a chemistry lab.

14. Household cleaners are the number one cause of death by poisoning; pesticides are the number two cause of death by poisoning.

15. Pesticides can remain for more than thirty years; inhalation can lead to nausea, coughing, breathing difficulties, depression, eye irritation and blurred vision, dizziness, twitching, convulsions, and more.

16. Canada Mortgage and Housing Corporation (CMHC) reports[146] that houses today are so airtight that most of the household chemicals build up because there is no place to go; 150 have been linked to birth defects, allergies, cancer,

and psychological abnormalities. (CMHC is Canada's premier provider of mortgage loan insurance and housing research.)

17. The most dangerous chemicals in household products are naphtha, a central nervous system depressant,[147] diethanolsamine, a liver poison, and/or chlorophenylphenol, a toxic metabolic stimulant.

18. The latest research from Greenpeace on toxins in clothing[148] revealed that fifty-two out of seventy-eight garments from fourteen global clothing brands sold in the UK and Europe tested positive for nonylphenol ethoxylates (NPEs), chemicals that are banned in clothing manufacturing. NPEs break down in water and metabolize into more toxic, less-biodegradable metabolites called nonylphenol (NP), a toxic, persistent substance that displays estrogenic properties, meaning that it can interfere with hormonal balance.

CHEMICAL TOXINS ARE EVERYWHERE

Whether we are talking about pesticides; chemicals put into the water deliberately, like chlorine and fluoride; or antibiotics that are used to keep animals from getting sick, which then end up on your dinner plate, keep in mind that all these chemicals are alien and dangerous to the organic life of the cell and therefore toxic to your body and brain.

They must be neutralized and removed.

It is impossible to determine where the chemicals originate, because they are so pervasive. A few examples of common sources of toxins may help illuminate the problem.

PESTICIDES

The pesticides used in commercial farming not only contaminate fruits and vegetables; they also seep into the water table. Pesticides inside your body could have come from products originating outside the United States, pesticide spraying around your home, or pesticides in the local school field.

XENOESTROGENS

The plastic bottles from which you drink beverages could be the source of xenoestrogens, which leak into the water or liquid and wreak havoc with your hormonal balance. Xenoestrogens mimic your own estrogens; therefore, the body cannot discriminate and protect itself. The fake estrogens hook up with molecules incorrectly, creating problems.

DIOXIN

Almost all of the dioxin inside your body comes from eating contaminated food. The contamination could have originated in the soil, in a local medical waste incinerator, or at a chlorine-based paper manufacturing plant.

ALUMINUM

Perhaps the most dangerous of all toxins are heavy metals, with aluminum at the top of the list because it is linked to many brain diseases. It appears that when overwhelmed with this metal, the body cannot get rid of it, and it ends up in places like the hippocampus, the brain's control center for memory and learning.

Aluminum is in your cookware, deodorant, medication, food, body care lotions, and even your drinking water. To be vigilant about this unwanted metal, know where it comes from and how it literally gets under your skin.

❖ **Cookware.** Most cooking pans and saucers are coated with aluminium. Even Teflon is coated. A better choice is to use stainless steel or cast iron and throw away all of your other cookware.

❖ **Medications.** Aluminum is present in most popular over-the-counter and prescription medicines like pain killers, anti-diarrhea drugs, and antacids. Antacids contain 200 milligrams of aluminium in a single tablet, ten times more than the acceptable limit per day.

❖ **Food.** Aluminum is in many processed foods like cheeses. It is used as an emulsifying agent in self-rising flour, nondairy creamers, and baking powder. Aluminium compounds are used in food additives, so you see various forms of it in cake mixes, chocolate mixes, coffee creamers like Coffee Mate, and ready-made dough.

❖ **Drinking water.** Fluoride is added to drinking water in the US, and in many countries, the water itself has high levels of aluminium. This becomes a highly toxic cocktail that appears to penetrate the blood-brain barrier, or BBB.(BBB is a separation of circulating blood from the brain designed to protect our brains from "foreign substances", while maintaining a constant environment).

❖ **Body care products.** You may see this ingredient in shampoo: aluminium laurel sulphate. In dandruff shampoos like Selsun Blue, you see the ingredient magnesium aluminium silicate. In antiperspirants, you see aluminium chlorhydrate

Most of us are not in the habit of reading labels for items that we have used for years or decades. Start reading labels. Watch out for aluminum in its various forms, and prevent the build up of heavy metals that could end up in your brain.

PARABENS

Parabens are used as preservatives in antiperspirants, cosmetics, and suntan lotion. Studies show that all parabens have estrogenic activity in human breast cells. Estrogenic activity can stimulate cancerous growths.

Dr Joseph Mercola talked about this in one of his weekly reports. He linked parabens to cancerous growths in human breast tissue. The culprit was antiperspirants and cosmetics. In the *Journal of Applied Toxicology*, which he cited, an editorial piece revealed that higher concentrations of parabens were found in the upper quadrants of the breast and surrounding area, the area where deodorants are applied.

If you are still not convinced about the enormous amount of chemical toxins that you are exposed to daily, refer to the chart below. It was created by the Dr. Mercola and his researchers and is available on the Mercola website. It is reprinted here in its entirety.[149]

Parabens	Heavily used preservatives in the cosmetic industry; used in an estimated 13,200 cosmetic and skin care products.	Studies implicate their connection with cancer because their hormone-disrupting qualities mimic estrogen and could disrupt your body's endocrine system.
Mineral Oil, Paraffin, and Petrolatum		These petroleum products coat the skin like plastic, clogging pores and creating a build-up of toxins. They can slow cellular development, *creating*

		earlier signs of aging. They're implicated as a suspected *cause of cancer. Plus, they can disrupt hormonal activity. When you think about black oil pumped from deep underground,* ask yourself why you'd want to put that kind of stuff on your skin.
Sodium laurel or lauryl sulfate (SLS), also known as sodium laureth sulfate (SLES)	Found in over 90 percent of personal care products! They break down your skin's moisture barrier, potentially leading to dry skin with premature aging. And because they easily penetrate your skin, they can allow other chemicals easy access.	SLS combined with other chemicals may become a "nitrosamine" – a potent carcinogen.
Acrylamide	Found in many facial creams.	Linked to mammary tumors.
Propylene glycol	Common cosmetic moisturizer and carrier for fragrance oils.	May cause dermatitis and skin irritation. May inhibit skin cell growth. Linked to kidney and liver problems.

Phenol carbolic acid	Found in many lotions and skin creams.	Can cause circulatory collapse, paralysis, convulsions, coma, and even death from respiratory failure.
Dioxane	Hidden in ingredients such as PEG,* polysorbates, laureth, ethoxylated alcohols. Very common in personal care products. *Polyethyleneglycol (PEG) products are likely to be contaminated with 1,4-dioxane, a carcinogen	These chemicals are often contaminated with high concentrations of highly volatile 1,4-dioxane that's easily absorbed through the skin. Its carcinogenicity was first reported in 1965, and later confirmed in studies including one from the National Cancer Institute in 1978. Nasal passages are considered extremely vulnerable, making it, in my opinion, a really bad idea to use these things on your face.
Toluene	May be very poisonous! Made from petroleum and coal tar... found in most synthetic fragrances.	Chronic exposure linked to anemia, lowered blood cell count, liver or kidney damage...May affect a developing fetus.

EMOTIONAL TOXINS

The last category of toxins is emotions. Although less understood, except in functional medicine, emotions are toxic to the body and mind. When you are upset or stressed, your body produces high levels of hormones. They may help you cope initially, but they must be removed, or they can disrupt your internal balance.

ARE YOU EXPERIENCING TOXIC OVERLOAD?

Are you experiencing toxic overload in your life, and does this toxicity create imbalances in your health landscape? It is our view, and the view of most functional medicine practitioners, that the body is overwhelmed with toxins that it must neutralize and eliminate.

A vacuum cleaner has a bag for collecting waste as the machine sucks up dirt and garbage from the floor. Picture what happens when the bag is full. It will bulge at the seams when it has taken in as much as it can. Your body is like this. Your liver and kidneys, the main conduits for detoxification, are constantly working to keep you out of harm's way by removing the onslaught of toxins.

We are not equipped to deal with the exponential increase in toxins. Our vacuum bag is likely full, and our detoxification systems are weakened and overloaded. The toxins stay in our body and in brain, and we are getting fatter (toxins are stored in adipose tissue) and sicker.

A recent study in Sweden showed a shocking 40 percent increase in dementia in the last five to seven years. Studies have shown that people with diseases of the brain, like Alzheimer's disease, have high concentrations of aluminum in their brain.[150]

Recall the conversation we had in Chapter 8 about acidic wastes and alkalinity: Acidic wastes favor cellular degeneration and promote the growth of bacteria. Toxins are a form of acidic wastes, the arch nemesis of superior health.

This is why you need to help your body detoxify. Without awareness of which toxins you are exposed to and without a health strategy to remove them, you are destined for disease, chronic illness, arthritis, or other forms of premature demise.

We believe that detoxification is an essential health strategy for twenty-first-century living. If done correctly, it can be like "emptying the garbage" and replacing your internal "vacuum bag."

The controversy about assisted detoxification is heated. We prefer that you learn the facts about your environment and decide whether assisted detoxification, also called cleansing (we refer to it as Assisted Detoxification Therapy or ADT), makes sense for you. You can then prioritize and incorporate this strategy into your health plan.

WHY IS DETOXIFICATION ESSENTIAL?

As the external environment becomes polluted, so does your internal environment; a cleansing health strategy enhances your natural detoxification system so you can get rid of dangerous accumulations of harmful toxins.

The overwhelming toxic burden is evident in the escalation of diseases that were once rare: everything from diabetes and coronary heart disease, impaired functions of the pancreas, and clogged arteries to brain diseases like dementia, Alzheimer's disease, and Parkinson's disease. Research shows that these diseases are occurring earlier and at alarming rates.

The awareness that we have a polluted environment, everything from our soil and our water to our food and our air brings us to the next critical question: What can we do to protect ourselves from these harmful chemicals, if they are everywhere?

PROPOSED SOLUTION

Toxic burden requires that you assist your detoxification processes with corrections in your daily eating habits, with conscientious, self-imposed control over toxic exposure, and/or implement an assisted therapy to support the body's detoxification chemistry.

ASSISTED DETOXIFICATION THERAPY (ADT)

We endorse ADT because we believe that our internal detoxification systems are no longer adequate for safely disposing of the toxic overload. We all need to eliminate or reduce the sources of toxins and increase toxin release.

Historically, almost all religions dealt with toxins through practices like fasting. The fast calls for a complete elimination of certain foods, like dairy, oils, and fats, (or meats during Lent- a doctrine of Christian spirituality) or abstaining from food after sundown (Ramadan- an Islamic obligation). These practices, followed for a period of two to three weeks or a month, allow the digestive system to relax and clean out the foods that create the most metabolic waste and stress. Once or twice a year, people who fast are able to "cleanse."

The food of the last century was not as polluted, not biogenetically modified, not full of preservatives, and not denatured of high-quality nutrients.

Fasting today, as opposed to the past, is practiced by fewer people and for shorter periods. There are other solutions to help your body cleanse itself of toxins. The simplest way is to implement the following practices for one or two weeks, three or four times each year, or one week per month:

1)   Increase your water intake, which in and of itself helps move toxins out of the body;

2) Eat or extract the juice (also called "juicing") from high-quality, raw vegetables and fruits;

3) Drink detox teas and juice, often available in health food stores;

4) Exercise to build up a sweat, or at least walk, every day while fasting or cleansing;

5) Find a sauna, and use it frequently.

If you find these practices too difficult to execute, eat or juice organic, high-quality, raw fruits and vegetables on a regular basis.

CHAPTER 10:

✡ ✡ ✡

HIGH-PERFORMANCE ACTION PLAN

"A goal is a dream with a deadline." —***Napoleon Hill***

"Let no feeling of discouragement prey upon you, and in the end you are sure to succeed." —***Abraham Lincoln***

STEP 9: CREATE YOUR HIGH-PERFORMANCE ACTION PLAN, STAY COMMITTED, AND REMEMBER THAT SUCCESS COMES ONE STEP AT A TIME.

Each person has DNA-specific bio-individuality. We are all unique; some of us love sports, others love dancing or swimming. We are differentiated by DNA markers, food preferences, entertainment choices, and likes and dislikes in every area of life. It is up to you to tailor your HP program and Action Plan to fulfil your dreams.

The guidelines we present will help you create your high-performance Action Plan. They help you develop a framework for establishing goals and action steps. Once you set up a daily, weekly, and monthly program, you can begin to create your new and improved HP lifestyle.

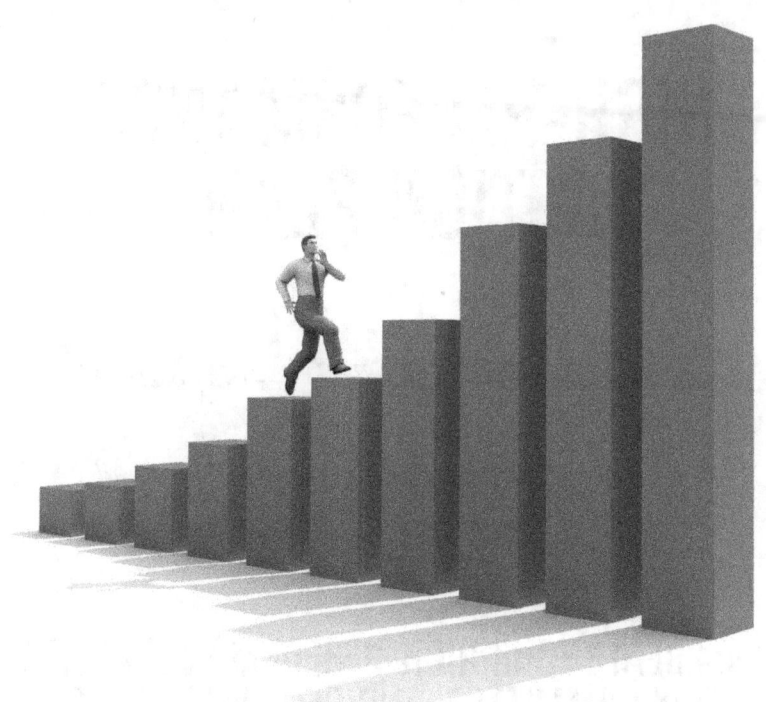

TEN STEPS

1 — START WITH THE TEN STEPS TO HIGH PERFORMANCE

Step 1. Understand that your ability achieve high performance is connected to your level of health. Decide that achieving superior health is a top priority now and for the rest of your life. Once you commit to this goal, make active choices to support this decision.

Step 2. Identify your baseline (current health status) and create simple, attainable coals divided into a specific timeframe for achievement (Action Plan). To attain any goal we set for ourselves, we must first develop a plan. The plan must have deadlines to keep us on track and motivated. Think of it as a journey from one side of a country to the other side. You need a map, where you can clearly identify which roads take you to the other side. Each road will have a number, and you can calculate how many hours you will drive and at which points you will stop and rest.

Your Action Plan will be your map. Once you know where you start the journey (baseline), and where you are going (goals), you can create markers for success.

Step 3. Become conscious of the body-brain connection.

The brain and body communicate as a two-way street. Emotions, stress, and fear can affect your physical body (headaches, backaches, and insomnia, to name a few). Likewise, physical exertion and nutrition can affect your brain (energetic or tired, anxious or optimistic, motivated or depressed).

For purposes of this book, we are interested in the connection between fuel, the gut, and the ability to function. The gut has more than one hundred million neurons; it is sometimes called "the second brain." This fact is often overlooked or underestimated, but the impact of the gut on the brain is well documented.

Step 4. Start with your head, and work your way down.

The head is the control center of your life; it controls thoughts and feelings, it processes information, it tells you when you are stressed, and it signals danger. It allows you to experience happiness, joy, and the exhilaration of achievement, pride, or a beautiful sunset. If your goal is to a achieve HP and a better life, invest in a better brain. Start with brain fuel, because it impacts the quality of your thoughts and feelings.

Step 5. Learn the basics for superior health or Cellular Energy Optimization (CEO). The fundamental principle of superior health is simple: optimize the performance of the cells in your body, which creates better functioning organs, systems, better balance, and better health. The basic requirements are high-quality water, air, sun, sleep, recharging, fuel, and exercise.

To achieve HP, put more emphasis on the basic fuel and energy supply for your brain and body and be vigilant about removing "energy bandits." These "bandits" can be people who absorb your time and energy. They are also the foods and toxins that deplete energy by using vitamins and minerals to metabolize (sugar) or remove dangerous substances (like mercury in tooth fillings, aluminum, and other heavy metals) without providing nutrients.

Step 6. Exercise daily. Physical activity (respiration and perspiration) generates vitality and energy, builds stamina, and improves brain performance.

Exercise affects the body and brain in numerous positive ways and must be included in any plan to achieve or maintain high performance. Perhaps most importantly, it helps keep the fluids in the blood moving, which brings in oxygen and moves out toxins. If toxins are not removed, they get stuck inside arteries and blood vessels and create conditions for inflammation and degenerative ailments (arthritis, cardiovascular deterioration). Ill health slows you down, detracts from focus, and depletes energy. High performers know that fitness is like an engine; it gives them constant energy so that they stay productive.

Studies show that people who exercise usually have better performance in a range of cognitive tasks versus non-exercisers. Other studies show that exercise improves longevity, etc.

Step 7. Make Choices that Maintain Balance. Superior health is balance. When you make conscious choices that help your body maintain key biological and psychological balances, your brain function, emotional responses, and health improve dramatically.

Balance, both biological and emotional, generates qualities that lead to high performance. Balance must be achieved in several areas for the body and mind to sustain optimal health:

1) Energy expended during the day is balanced by sleep at night, when the body does cellular repair work and detoxifies.

2) Stress must be balanced by renewal therapies that restore energy and a positive outlook.

3) Biochemical balance is the correct ratio of nutrients, like omega 6 and omega 3 from fish and olive oil, or a high intake of vegetables, that in turn yield the optimal alkaline-to-acid ratio to sustain health.

4) Emotional balance is maintained when you have strong and rewarding relationships with key family members and/or friends.

Step 8. Beware of toxins, and use detoxification methods to assist natural detoxification. Detoxification is no longer an optional health strategy. It is necessary, in your journey for superior health, to become more aware of what can help you nutritionally *and* what can harm you. Toxins can come from the food you eat, the liquids you drink (artificial sweeteners, for example), the dry cleaning chemicals and body lotions absorbed into your skin, the mercury fillings in your teeth, and the fluoride in water. If you lived in the nineteenth or first half of the twentieth century, this strategy might not be part of the discussion.

We are exposed to six million pounds of mercury and more than two billion pounds of other toxins each year. The Environmental Working Group reports that the average newborn baby has 287 known toxins in his or her umbilical cord—a frightening but thought-provoking fact.

Foods are no longer grown on pesticide-free farms but are processed, contaminated, and denatured, leaving them devoid of essential nutrients, and worse, tainted with residual chemicals. Cattle and poultry are not raised to roam or fed grass and seeds (rich in omega 3s, a powerful brain fuel) but are raised commercially and fed antibiotics to keep them from getting sick. Industrially raised animals are not fed grass but soy (which reduces omega 3 and raises the intake of pro-inflammatory omega 6), because it is cheaper.

Step 9. Create your Action Plan, stay committed, and remember that success comes one step at a time. A realistic game plan for improving health should have the eight components explained below.

Each component has an opposite aspect, much as a battery has a negative and positive charge. They represent the balance in your system. Understanding these balances and applying them will help you see the patterns in your daily life.

PHYSIOLOGICAL

In (Nutrition/Toxins)	⟷	Out (Detoxification)
Work, Exercise	⟷	Sleep, Rest, Restore

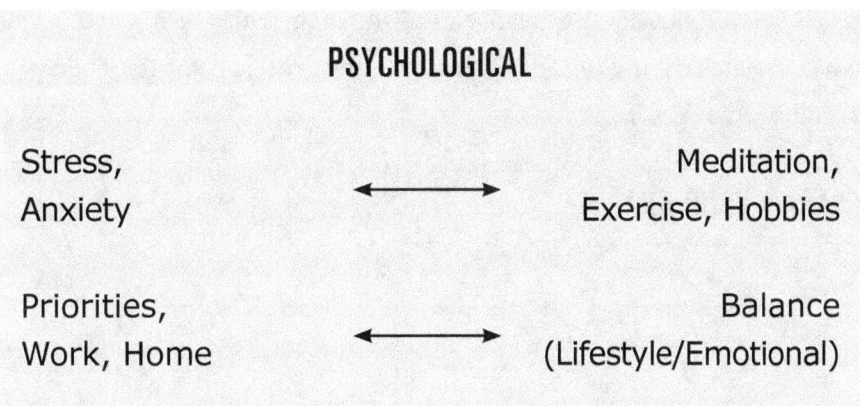

PSYCHOLOGICAL

Stress, Anxiety ⟷ Meditation, Exercise, Hobbies

Priorities, Work, Home ⟷ Balance (Lifestyle/Emotional)

Step 10. Develop new systems and habits. Consciously integrate them into your daily routines to assist you in achieving superior health and a high-performance lifestyle.

Review the steps to identify the strong and weak links in your health armor. For example, if your weight is not what you need it to be, this can be one of your priorities. If your weight is fine but your stress is through the roof, learn what cranks up your stress and what response mechanisms you can put in place to reduce it.

Once you have identified your weakest links, focus on the one or two most important ones, the ones that interfere with your quality of life and focus.

2 — WRITE DOWN YOUR GOALS: PREPARE YOUR MIND

Go back to the beginning of this book. If you wrote down your goal and attached a picture of what your goal represents and five things that motivate you, take out that paper, reread it, adjust it, and make sure that you have the same objectives as when you started.

If you did not do this exercise, read the suggestions below, and decide what you are striving for now. To achieve any goal, it helps to understand it and write it down.

CLARIFY YOUR GOAL

The first step in writing an Action Plan is to clarify your goal.

- What outcome do you hope to achieve? Can you define it with words or visualize it (create a new company; start a new business, become a more-involved parent, etc.)?
- How will you know that you have achieved it (how will you feel, what will change in your world, what are the markers)?
- What makes the goal measurable (what steps, strategies, or outcomes will you see)?
- What constraints do you have (time, money, resources), and can you improvise alternatives to remove the obstacles? If you cannot find appropriate alternatives, your goal is not realistic. Rethink the process again, or be innovative in overcoming road blocks. Innovating is another characteristic of HP.

We recommend re-reading this book and giving yourself time to prepare your mind. Review the balances described in Step 9. See which balances are not working for you, and set a goal. If you are set with your goals, break each goal into subgoals, and write a list of actions, strategies, and routines to implement or change to achieve them.

For example, if your goal is to lose twenty pounds in twelve weeks, your three subgoals might be to increase water intake 50 percent to ten glasses a day, get at least thirty minutes of exercise a day, and replace pasta meals with lean or nonmeat protein and vegetable meals twice a week.

If your goal is to reduce stress, find two activities to incorporate into your daily schedule that provide an outlet for stress. This can be resuming an old hobby (like fishing on the weekend), a thirty-minute massage each morning, or ten minutes of meditation each day.

3 — IDENTIFY YOUR LIST OF ACTION STEPS

Write a list of steps needed to take to achieve your goal, and think of as many different options as possible.

On another sheet of paper, write more ideas about how you can achieve your goal without judging the merit of each action. Prioritize your good ideas and action steps, and strike the unnecessary ones from the list. Mark the steps that you feel are the most effective and realistic. Identify which steps are critical and highlight them, and identify which ones can be eliminated without seriously affecting your outcome.

ORGANIZE YOUR LIST INTO A SEQUENCE

Decide on the order of your action steps by looking at the critical steps (the ones you highlighted). For each action, determine if there are other steps that should be completed. Rearrange your actions and ideas into a sequence that makes sense.

DECIDE TO ACHIEVE

You now have a ladder of action steps to reach your goal. Repeat this process for each goal. Make a decision that you will achieve your goal and that you will be able to make the changes that are conducive to your HP journey.

The goal-setting process is an essential first step. It creates the destination in your map. Once you figure out your starting point and your goal, the action steps and the road map to HP health become more visible.

4 — DETERMINE WAYS TO MONITOR EXECUTION AND MEASURE SUCCESS

Let's examine losing weight again, as this is usually one of the obstacles that block superior health. Weight loss can also be one of three goals that you identify as part of your grand plan to become a high performer. For simplicity's sake, let's say you want to lose twenty pounds in three months. You listed your action steps, which may include three changes in your meals, an exercise program, and reducing alcohol.

You could attach a measurement for each action, like burning calories while walking. To do this, you can buy a pedometer or a Nike Fuel Band, a universal metric of activity that tracks your all-day activity and motivates you to do more. Let's say that you set a goal of 1,000 calories burned per week from walking. You could divide the goal into five days. This would enable you to be more conscious of how much exercise you get in a day, and you can get creative in how to achieve your "burn calories" goal.

Know that 3,500 calories equals about 1 pound, or half a kilo, of fat. You need to burn 3,500 calories more than you take in to lose 1 pound. We do not recommend counting food calories, because we believe the focus should be on quality nutrients and less on quantity. When you are focused on quantity, you enter a negative zone—what you are cutting back, what you are *not* eating, and which foods are high in calories (even though they may be high on the health barometer).

Having said this about calories, we do understand that some people are motivated by measurements of success, and burning calories while exercising can be a powerful motivator if you track your progress daily or weekly. Although you should avoid focusing on calories and focus on nutrients, it *is* helpful to understand what calories you burn when you exercise if weight management or loss is one of your goals. There are several online sites that can give you guidelines in this area, like the Mayo Clinic. (http://www.mayoclinic.com/)

Another approach is to make the goal more generic. Do two activities during the day that burn calories for a total of at least one hour.

These kinds of measures can be set up in a daily, weekly, or monthly planner.

If strengthening your stress management skills is your goal, observe how many coping mechanisms you have in your tool trunk and if they serve you sufficiently. If you need to improve this area, become conscious of your triggers, and find new techniques that give you more satisfying results.

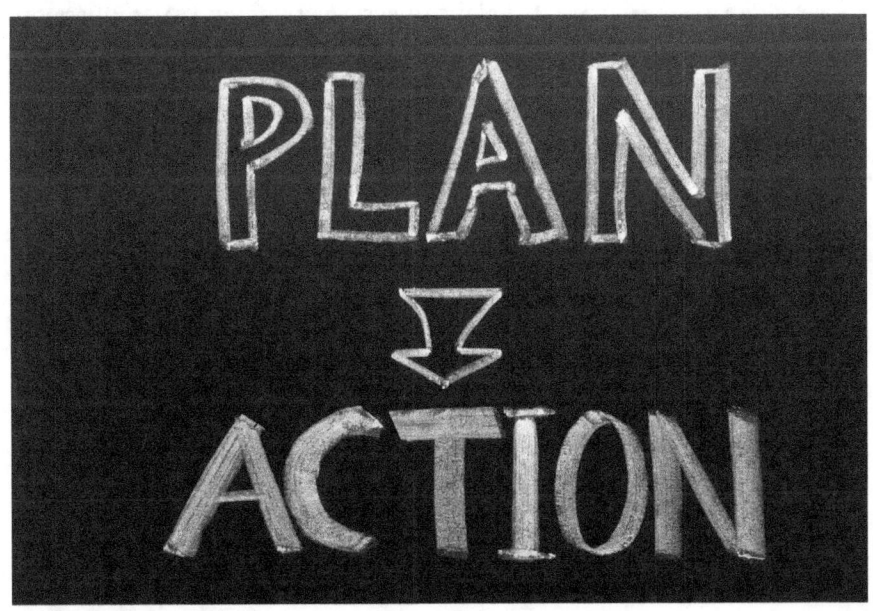

5 — READY, ON YOUR MARK, GET SET, ACTION!

If you follow these guidelines, you should be able to create your action plan. Here is an example.

Goal statement: Improve my energy levels at work and home by losing twenty pounds in three months so that I feel less tired throughout the day, more energetic on the weekends, and more productive at work.

ACTIONS

- Learn what foods are healthy, and identify my favorites in each category.
- Increase the number of healthy foods I eat at each meal.
- Cut out three anti-nutrients: less coffee, no alcohol, and no trans fats.
- Plan my meals so that I balance macro nutrients and micronutrients.
- Make a new food list, find an appropriate store, and shop for items.
- Set aside time to prepare and eat healthy meals.
- Schedule three hours of exercise a week (thirty to forty-five minutes each morning).

MEASURES

- Eat a healthy breakfast of fruits or proteins every day.
- Eat five servings of vegetables during the day: three at lunch, two at dinner.
- Eat one salad every day.
- Replace junk food with high-energy nuts, seeds, and organic protein bars.

- Find my weakest spot in terms of diet, and actively seek a substitute (e.g., sweets for my sweet tooth that are healthier).
- Walk to work, and schedule thirty minutes of aerobic activity four times a week.
- Have a checklist for each action step, and go ten days in a row without lapsing into bad habits.
- Repeat twenty days in a row without lapsing until I hit three months.

SCHEDULE YOURSELF EVERY DAY

Even the most organized people fail because they underestimate the commitment and tenacity it takes to root out entrenched, routine behavior. Do you start each morning with several cups of coffee just to get going? Do you have an identifiable pattern in your morning? Does it include a routine you have identified for HP like drinking more water, exercising, or doing something that relaxes your mind? Chances are that if you identified your weak links, you need to find ways to break the patterns that keep you in the "old mold." Carve out time to work on routines that create the "new mold" of you.

Schedule time for yourself. If you have an assistant, have him or her put you on the calendar. Have a code for it if you need this camouflage in order to create space on your calendar. Write yourself in at least sixty minutes each day. This can be thirty minutes in the morning and evening, or twenty-minute increments, or whatever works for you.

You may need to adjust your entire day. Decide what you are going to work on every day during this time. Is it your exercise program? Developing a new hobby? Changing your refrigerator into a high-powered fuel supply station?

Schedule time for yourself as though you were meeting with your most important client or as if you were a doctor about to perform surgery. It is something you prioritize or it is not. We are usually successful in the things we prioritize, so listen to the little voice in your head when the world around you runs interference. If something unavoidable derails your schedule, get the "train back on track" as soon as possible.

6 — PREPARE A REALISTIC TIMELINE

When is it realistic to begin a program that will require you to make some interesting or even drastic changes in your routines? Realistically, when can you start?

We advise taking out a calendar and looking at the weeks and months ahead. Without looking for cheesy excuses, make sure that you have nothing major in your path that might derail your path. For example, if you are going through a messy divorce, renovating your house, or gearing up for an annual shareholder's meeting, this is not a good time to start.

You need to be able to focus and stay motivated and committed to your outcomes. On the other hand, if you have a shareholders meeting in two months or are going to a wedding in three months (and you are not the person planning the wedding), your action plan can be motivating.

Once you establish a start date, determine how many weeks you need to achieve your goal. Start with a short-term plan and a long term-plan. The short-term plan should be a realistic goal that you can achieve in twelve weeks. A realistic timeframe for achieving one or two of your goals can motivate you to continue.

The long-term goal can be one that you accomplish in six months to a year.

SAMPLE TIMETABLE

Week 1: Learn about healthy foods; make a list of your favorites to include in meals. Decide what type of exercise to include in your program, and plan the execution (join a gym, find a tae kwon do studio, etc.).

Week 2: Develop a template for meal planning, and figure out the best way to execute your plan (30 percent take-out high-quality meals, 70 percent meals cooked at home, etc.)

Week 3: Identify foods that are low in nutrition, and replace them with ones with high nutrition value (particularly micro nutrient rich foods found in vegetables).

Week 4: **Start.** *You will not succeed unless you show up for your own life plan.*

ACTION PLAN

GOAL_____

Objectives (List of Outcomes you hope to achieve)	Tasks (What do you need to do to achieve your objectives) Action steps:	Success Criteria (How can you measure your success)	Time Frame (When do you need to achieve the tasks)	Resources (What Resources do you need for each task)

7 — IDENTIFY ADVOCATES AND CHEERLEADERS

The job of achieving HP is a commitment. Recognize that not everyone will support your goals, so identify your detractors, and minimize your exposure to negativity. Find the people who love and support you in your endeavor to improve your mind, body, and performance. Let them know that you are working on a plan and that you need them "on the sidelines" to cheer you on. Most advocates are great when enlisted for support. Enlist a friend, a colleague, a wife, or a husband. Even better, find someone who wants to join you, so that you have a support system and a partner in your HP plan.

You not only need commitment and time, but you need to spend time finding the right strategies for succeeding. For example, if you do not regularly drink water, how do you correct this? Falling back into old habits is easy because you get used to your patterns over a period of time. Breaking routines and developing new ones therefore is harder than you think.

Since at least one of the authors (Type A, overachieving, and previously chronically dehydrated) can attest, it is imperative that you figure out how to drink more water. Start with water stations. Place bottles of Evian or your favorite water in several places with a glass nearby. Take sips throughout the day at each station, or drink half a glass, until you achieve your goal of ten to twelve glasses. Drink one full glass twenty minutes before eating, as this helps curb your appetite. Remind yourself too that wine, soda, coffee and teas (containing sugars and/or caffeine) are not suitable alternatives to water.

If you want fitness, try hiring a life or physical fitness coach. If you want improved nutrition, find new restaurants and organic-oriented supermarkets, and use your scheduled "me time" for discovering new delights.

IDENTIFY NEGATIVE INFLUENCES AND PROTECT YOURSELF

You can have "energy robbers" and "people parasites"—people who take up your time and energy, depleting you of the energy you need for other priorities. Find the systems that eliminate some or all of your energy thieves.

Thieves can also come in the form of what you do, who you know, and what you eat and drink. Identify these behaviors and choices, and decide on alternatives. For example, if you have wine with lunch, cocktails before dinner, and wine with your meal, wake up and smell the alcohol: Alcohol, we repeat, is not a health food. It is an anti-nutrient, and too much is dangerous to your health and your ability to achieve an HP lifestyle.

If you find that you are guilty of the stimulant-stress-stimulant pattern, decrease the coffee, increase the water and exercise, and add a green drink every day for a power boost.

8 — MIRROR, MIRROR ON THE WALL

Can you hold up the mirror and see which behaviors you have adopted that do not serve you? Write down five of them. What can you do to break the behaviors? What can you do to replace the behavior patterns?

Make another column, and write five alternate actions that can, over time, become substitute behaviors. Draw an arrow between the poor habit and the better behavior. It can take anywhere from 18 to 254 days to change an old habit and reshape a new pattern, according to recent research published in the July 16, 2009 European Journal of Social Psychology. The variance, according to the research, is linked primarily to the magnitude of the habit. If it is a simple habit, say, not eating a donut with coffee in the morning, and having a piece of fruit instead, the habit could take a month to reshape. For something more ambitious, like doing 50 sit-ups before breakfast, or quitting smoking, it might take up to a year.[151]

Habits can form through repetition, so they become automatic, or they can develop as a response to an enjoyable event that triggers the brain's "reward" centers. The latter can be harmful to our health, because the routines become inescapable, like overeating, smoking, drug or alcohol abuse, gambling and even compulsive use of computers and social media.[152]

We become comfortable in our habits. Like a pair of old jeans, they slip on easily, and you can be emotionally attached to them. Pleasure based habits in particular, are difficult to break because they stimulate the pleasure seeking area of the brain, which then releases dopamine, a chemical which then reinforces our desire to seek the same pleasure (thereby creating the impetus to repeat the behavior and forming a habit).

But here is the good news: According to Dr Roy Baumeister, a psychologist at Florida State University, "Humans are much better than any other animal at changing and orienting our behavior toward long-term goals, or long term benefits." He concluded from his research on decision-making and willpower that "self-control is like a muscle...you can improve your self-control by doing exercises over time. Any regular act of self-control will gradually exercise your 'muscle' and make you stronger."[153]

If your habits do not serve you, look at them for what they are: goal blockers, energy thieves, disrupters of focus, and motivational leeches. Start replacing them with higher quality actions.

For example, if you start your day on the computer and then can't find time to exercise, start your day with a brisk walk or an exercise class.

9 — LEVERAGE POSITIVE MOTIVATION

Look at the photo you are using as your motivation visual. Maybe it's a photo of you when you started working and your motivation and enthusiasm were at their highest. Maybe it's a photo of you with a fish on a dock or a sailboat, when fishing was one of your passions. Maybe it's a picture of someone you admire who is a successful high performer, and your goal is to become more like this person.

Create a strong visual to reinforce your motivation. Motivation is a source of fusion energy: it can propel you toward a desired outcome, and it is a positive force. It is the "I can do this" mantra in your head. In contrast, willpower is temporary and comes from a negative energy ("I will *not* do this" or "I will *stop* doing that").

Another approach is to leverage a specific activity or event. Say that you have a specific activity that is motivating—you have been invited to be a speaker on a TV program, or you are chairing an important board meeting. These can be motivations. Whatever it is, use it!

Think about to how great you will feel once you feel lighter, more energetic, more rested, and more "on fire." Leverage these feelings every time you think about why you are doing something different from the old you. It is the right path to the new you.

10 — START

Start! It sounds simple, but starting can be the second hardest step in your health journey. The hardest step is sticking with the changes that you want to make.

When you were learning to ride a bicycle, falling off was part of the learning process. Getting back on the bicycle and hanging in there until you got your balance and your rhythm, the pedals rotating automatically, was the hardest part.

This is why we recommend realistic goals and timelines and urge you to create motivational tools to stay focused on the results you want.

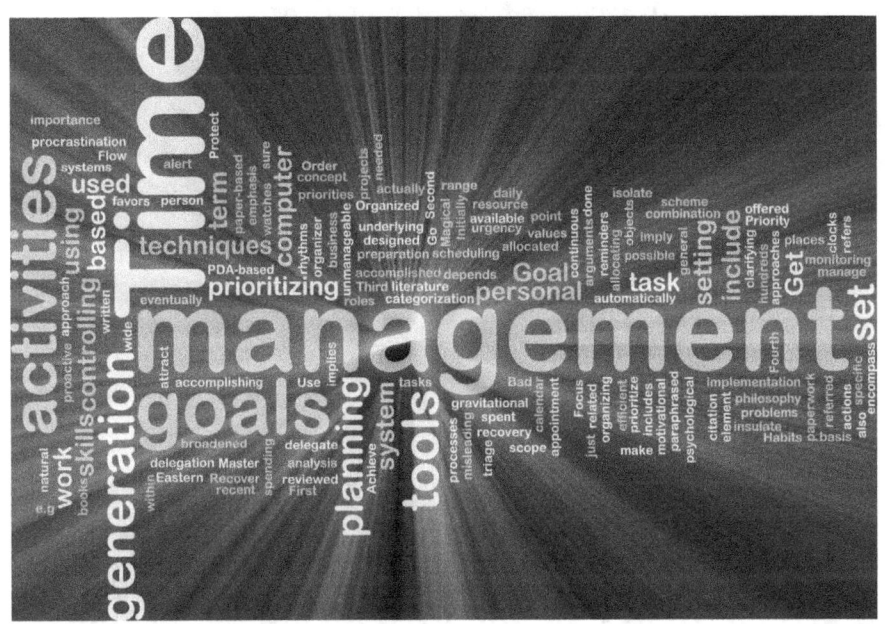

CHAPTER 11:

✧ ✧ ✧

SYSTEMS AND HABITS

"The critical ingredient is getting off your butt and doing something. It's as simple as that. A lot of people have ideas, but there are few who decide to do something about them now. Not tomorrow. Not next week. But today. The true entrepreneur is a doer, not a dreamer." —**Nolan Bushnell**

"We are what we repeatedly do. Excellence then,
is not an act, but a habit." —Aristotle

"We're worn into grooves by Time and by our habits. In the end, these
grooves are going to show whether we've been second rate or champions,
each in his way in dispatching the affairs of every day. By choosing
our habits, we determine the grooves into which Time will wear us;
and these are grooves that enrich our lives and make for ease of mind,
peace, happiness and achievement." —Frank B. Gilberth

STEP 10: DEVELOP NEW SYSTEMS AND HABITS. CONSCIOUSLY INTEGRATE THEM INTO YOUR DAILY ROUTINES TO ASSIST YOU IN ACHIEVING SUPERIOR HEALTH AND A HIGH-PERFORMANCE LIFESTYLE.

Ask yourself, "How much do I want to succeed in becoming a high performer?"

What is your motivation? Is it that you want to become an industry leader, the top performer at your company, a better husband, parent, teacher, salesperson, artist, actor, or manager? Do you simply want to achieve superior health? No matter what your motivation is, make sure that you are okay with it. Decide that superior health is your top priority, and make choices that support that decision. It sounds easy, but it's not.

Reengineering your habits and routines until they serve your purpose can be challenging. More often than not, you have habits that get in the way of what you are trying to achieve. Remember that success comes one step at a time. Be patient, and remind yourself that it takes anywhere from eighteen to two hundred and fifty four days to shake off an old routine and implement one that fits your new image and lifestyle.

SYSTEMS TO STAY MOTIVATED

- **Write it down!** Write your goal concisely, and print it out five times on a small but readable piece of paper. (You can use a photo or picture, if you are more visually oriented.) Put the paper where you can see it every day: on your bathroom mirror, on your laptop, on the door of your refrigerator, or on the door as you leave your house. Seeing it will remind you of your intention throughout the day as you dodge temptations and old habits.

- **Use photos and visuals to reinforce your image of what you will achieve, and look at them often.** Create a vision board, a simple cork board with visual representations of your goals in different categories using photos, magazine cut-outs,, words, or anything that helps your mind picture your goal and stay on point.

- **Tell three people.** Identify people who are positive and who support you. Let their enthusiasm and support be contagious.

- **Integrate the plan into your work environment.** If you are in a position of authority or are just persuasive and innovative, you can organize this:
  - Invite speakers, trainers, and other professionals to speak on health and fitness issues.
  - Create a contest, for example, who can lose the most weight in a sixty-day period, supported by speakers and information.
  - Challenge a competitor or a supplier with a contest related to fitness or a competition that requires regular exercise.

- Create an interdepartmental contest to get different groups of people involved. If the contest goal is aligned with your personal goal, you will have more "wind beneath your wings" when it comes to succeeding.

- **Hire a professional.** This is one of the surest ways to stay motivated, because it involves finding someone who can crack the whip when it needs cracking. If you are lazy when it comes to exercise, a trainer at your local gym can help you stay on track. If nutrition is your weak spot, seek a professional who can guide you with menu selection (often a personal trainer can guide you in this). If you need an all-around makeover, find a life coach.

- Life coaching is a burgeoning industry, and it should be easy to find someone qualified. Check references and look for referrals.

- **Remind yourself.** One of the keys to achieving your goals is to remind yourself of what you want to achieve. Willpower depletes energy, because you constantly remind yourself of what you do *not* want to do. Motivation works with positive energy: you are striving to achieve something (better health, better life, better job, more money). and because it is positive and strong, this energy can be harnessed to achieve your goals.

- **Focus your mind on what you want, and avoid ANTs.** Remember what Daniel Amen said about ANTs, automatic negative thoughts. Crush them. Achieving goals happens by focusing on what you want, and what you want will trump everything else. Amen used a picture of his grandchild as his screensaver. It was a constant reminder of why he worked so hard. What do you use as your screensaver? Understand and value the choices you will be making in the process that gets you to where you want to be and what you want to look and feel like.

- **Have fun!** The easiest way to stay motivated is to have fun. No plan can succeed unless there is a component of fun, so find ways to stimulate your fun barometer.
- Motivation, not willpower, is the key to success.

SYSTEMS FOR LEARNING

Let's go back to what we said about flying a plane. Pilots require a great deal of education as part of their training; they are not taken off the street and handed a license to fly. It takes education and lots of practice, coaching, and a desire to succeed.

Becoming the pilot of your health "plane" requires the same work. Educate yourself continuously so that you can become better in the short term and long term. You may need training from specialists (coaches, trainers, nutritionists, doctors) who have expertise in areas in which you may need help. You may need coaching so that you can identify your weaker skills and learn how to improve them. Although it may come as a surprise to some, to attain superior health, you need practice, and lots of it.

If you are self-motivated, reread this book from time to time; use it as a starter kit and a reference. Here are some further suggestions:

- **Enroll in a course at your local college.** Adult education is a way of "killing two birds with one stone." You get to increase your knowledge about an area you are interested in (cooking, nutrition, or scuba diving, whatever jazzes your synapses), and at the same time, you push away conditions like Alzheimer's diseases by keeping your mind alert. Make it fun, and make it one of your goals.
- **Find people who you know are into health, and start picking their brains.** They are fit, they skip the bagels and donuts

and opt for oatmeal with blueberries, and they go to the gym frequently. Ask them what they eat and why. They can fill you in on all sorts of interesting information.

- **Subscribe to a health magazine.** *Men's Health, Women's Health*, and other publications can expand your horizons on health issues.
- **Read three new books on a subject related to your health or high-performance goals**. If you are curious about other high performers, read a biography of someone who achieved great success, or stick with a classic like *Think and Grow Rich*. If you want to focus on motivation, find a self-help book on it. If psychoneuroimmunology floats your boat, go to a bookstore and find books on the subject. Don't get too excited, buy five books, and not read any of them. They cannot "talk to you" when they sit on your bookshelf or downloaded in your Kindle. Find one or two books, and add reading them into your Action Plan.
- **Ask your life coach and personal trainer for advice.** These are professionals who make it their business to help people reach their goals in fitness, health, business, and life.
- **Practice, practice, practice.** To get good at something, you need practice. It is the same with superior health. Practice turns what is new and unfamiliar into something comfortable and automatic. Practice health every day to become good at it.

SYSTEMS FOR ORGANIZATION

Start with the place that most needs structure and renovation. In the quest for HP, it is usually the kitchen, your office, or place of work.

- **What to buy, what to eat: flirt with yourself**

THE PREP WEEK: WHAT DO YOU LIKE TO EAT?

Make a list of the foods you like to eat, find the foods that are energy thieves, and create a good replacement list. Take a good week or two to try the foods from the "good guy" list. Find a sufficient quantity so that when you begin your HP plan, you have enough selection to migrate toward healthier eating. The foods on this list (which will be a continuous process) are what you need to put in your refrigerator and cupboard. You will have a "To Buy" list (high nutrition) and a "Poison" list (energy thieves).

- **Set up your criteria for food and meal selection.** Establish your criteria for eating healthy. For example, if you eat toast in the morning, make sure you eat multigrain toast. If you do not like salad, look for vegetable dishes that you can buy or make that taste good. Keep trying until you find substitutes you like. Eating healthy can be a challenge when you are surrounded by unhealthy choices, so stay on point and enlist your creativity to stay motivated. Rely on friends, family, colleagues and media resources for good habits; you can usually find worthwhile suggestions.
- **Restructure your kitchen.** It is time to get serious about improved health and fitness, and your refrigerator needs to reflect this. Keep salad, washed and ready to eat, in a storage container that keeps it fresh. Buy fruits and vegetables that you like to eat, but experiment with others. Keep high-quality sources of lean protein and vegetable protein (like tofu) in your refrigerator to create meals with or snack on. Shop organic whenever possible, so that you can keep the toxin level down and the nutrient level up.
- **Expand your repertoire of fruit, vegetable, and complex carbs.** Experiment with tastes, textures, and satisfaction in your arsenal of antioxidant, immune-building, disease-busting,

energy-enhancing foods. Try new dishes at restaurants, and go home and recreate them. Find new take-out places, and knock yourself out trying dishes that meet the criteria you have set up.

- **Develop water stations.** Any HP plan must include increasing water intake. To drink ten glasses a day (add two for every cup of coffee or caffeinated drink, including cola), keep three large bottles at "water stations." Make the stations near or in places you frequent during the day. If you spend most of your time at work, keep one bottle on or below your desk, another where you relax, watch television, or work on your computer, and anotherin your bedroom.

- **Schedule your day, every day, to include at least three health practices**. During the first week, you might plan and prep your schedule, meal options, and kitchen. In the second week, it may be learning an antistress routine, getting a massage, and taking the stairs in your office building instead of the elevator. The third week, it may be going to a new restaurant, trying a new class at the gym, or ordering a health drink from a local vendor.

If exercise is lacking in your routine, create a realistic program. Schedule a fifteen-minute walk, and work your way up to thirty minutes during the month. If your diet does not include enough vegetables, figure out a strategy for increasing this component in your meal plan (eat a green salad or schedule time to shop at an organic food store).

As you get healthier, your energy will increase. As this happens, challenge yourself. It is characteristic of high performers.

Invigorate your schedule by including new things. Once you have mastered a healthy practice, move on. This will keep you from getting bored. Get creative. If you have implemented a strong schedule and followed it for sixty days, try a new routine. Organize your work day to incorporate one to two new health practices each week. For example, if you have exercised consistently for three months, try a new class like tai chi, zumba dance aerobics, yoga, or martial arts. If you ate Caesar salads every day for lunch, go wild at a Japanese restaurant, and try seaweed or an avocado salad.

SYSTEMS FOR NUTRITIONAL UPGRADES

- **Employ a daily or weekly checklist to monitor your nutrition intake.** Once you know what is high-quality fuel for your brain and body, you can monitor how it rejuvenates your energy. Make a list of what you want to incorporate into your diet (alkaline fruits and vegetables, high-quality protein, etc.).

- **Make a list of foods and beverages that you know serve your goal and foods to avoid; use it or give it to the right person.** Never completely eliminate the "bad" foods until you are confident that you have replaced them with a better or equally satisfying option. You must be able to eat, occasionally, the foods you love. The trick is to keep reducing your intake of inferior-quality options by finding satisfying alternatives.

Use the list you have developed on a regular basis, at least at the beginning of your Action Plan. If you are not the person who shops and prepares meals, give the list to the person who does. Make sure that the person supports your goal and accommodates (rather than sabotages) your requests.

- **Be on the lookout for high-quality snacks.** They are the best ways to soothe the transition from junk to high quality. Try different options until you find something you like. Whole Foods and other health stores usually carry an assortment of energy bars, for example. Try different nuts and seeds. You can even create a montage of dried fruits, nuts, and seeds or buy a bag at a store like a Trader Joe's.

- **Find a reputable health expert online that you can follow**. There are many websites that offer advice on how to get healthy. Check them out, and adopt one or two suggestions. Check the sites often.

- **Work on your weakest links**. For example, if white foods are a big part of your repertoire, this exercise will be tough. Start with substitution. If you eat a lot of pasta, switch to whole-grain pasta. If you eat bread at restaurants, ask for a plate of olives or order a munchable appetizer like edamame or grilled vegetables. Too much sugar in your world? Get stevia at your health store. Replace white sugar with a healthy alternative.

❖ If you can't live without bread, switch to bread made with healthier grains, and eat brown rice. Brown rice is a slow-burning carb that releases energy slowly.

❖ If your beverage consumption is weak, implement the "drink more water" strategy first. Water will fill you up. Drink one cup of water twenty minutes before meals.

❖ If you find water boring compared to fizzy favorites, find a fruit tea that appeals to your taste buds and make it cold. Switch to carbonated water with lime and lemon until you get the hang of drinking more water.

Upgrade your fuel, and go for high octane. In the Notes section at the back of this book, we offer a list of the food fuels that give you the highest quality nutrition. If you are going to become an HP, master this part of your program. Get rid of your old programming; it no longer serves you. Upgrade your nutritional operating system so that you can think smarter, act smarter, and have the energy of an Olympic athlete.

Scratch routines that work against you, and replace them with routines that serve your goals. If you start your day with coffee, cut back. Coffee first thing in the morning is like pressing on the accelerator while your car is parked in the garage. When you wake up, your body is still detoxifying. Assist it, don't work against it. Start with water, and drink as much as you can. In the second hour, eat fruit, or drink a fruit smoothie. Delay your coffee until late morning. This is in itself a healthier habit.

If you drink too much diet soda, replace every other diet drink with water. Sodas have high fructose corn syrup and/or sugar substitutes (like aspartame), which create toxins in your body. Be conscious about what you are trying to achieve. The body and brain need water to flush out toxins.

SYSTEMS FOR EXERCISE

Exercise is your elixir for youthful energy, immunity, and detoxification. Work it into your schedule.

Figure out what you like to do, and do it. If you do not have a regular exercise program, start one. Explore your options, and they can include the things you like to do or used to like to do: tennis, racquetball, swimming, jogging, tae kwon do, dancing, or walking.

Once you identify your options, decide which form of exercise suits you or which one you wish to develop. Make a choice and a commitment. If you love dancing, find a place, and a partner, to make this happen (a local dance studio, evenings with your spouse or friends). If this does not work on a consistent basis, enroll in a class. If all else fails, find your favorite CDs, and schedule a dance-a-thon in your living room. If you need the freedom to express yourself, pick a time when no one is around.

If none of these options make sense to you, start with twenty-minute walks. Increase the speed gradually until you are taking a brisk walk, and then increase the time. The trick is to find the time. Schedule yourself accordingly.

- **Get off your BUT.** One of my favorite expressions, coined by self-help guru and inspirational therapist Sean Stephenson, is "get off your but." We all have our "buts," and they are especially noticeable when avoiding something you need to do. You may find yourself saying, "I would like to exercise but"...

  - I don't have time
  - I work long hours
  - I run a company
  - I run a business
  - I travel too much
  - The gym is far from where I live
  - My schedule is too tight
  - I have to make a deadline this month
  - I have to meet my quota this month
  - I am working on a big presentation
  - I hate working out at the gym
  - I can't find a class I like

- I have to lose weight first
- I am waiting for a package
- My tooth hurts
- I have to feed the cat

Get the picture? Do you have a but?

If you are going to succeed at anything that is difficult, find a way to get off your but, and catch yourself when you are but-ting.

- **Enlist a partner who shares your goal.** Having someone to exercise with makes exercise fun. Pick an activity like biking, walking, canoeing, or going to the gym, and find someone who will join you.

- **Incorporate physical activity into your workday.** If you are an overstressed, overscheduled executive, have meetings with colleagues while taking a walk. Schedule your next meeting with your colleague, associate, or business partner while walking in a park or on a gym track.

- **Measure your progress.** Do this each day or week, and reward yourself once you are satisfied that you have earned your reward. If you need to run around a track three times a week, keep a record, and surprise yourself.

- **Pushing beyond your limits helps you achieve what seemed impossible, so shatter your limits.** If you are a person who enjoys competition, compete with yourself. Have a measureable goal, and surpass it over the medium term. You will make yourself crazy if you outdo yourself every day, so set a weekly goal of, say, five miles of running or walking—then five and a half. This will inspire you to compete with yourself.

- **Dare to have fun.** Just as with learning, studies show that you are more successful when you are having fun. Shift your attitude. Find activities that are engaging while they burn calories. Golfing could be great if you didn't drive around in a golf cart. You can start by walking the front nine, and reward yourself by using the golf cart on the back nine. You are moving more and incorporating a good sweat into one of your favorite activities.

- **Get it done, and benefit from increased oxygen to your brain.** Bring oxygen to your brain with exercise in the morning. The higher the oxygen content to your brain, the better your thought process and decision making, so think about that when you are preparing for an early-morning meeting.

Walking is simple and easy to do anywhere. If you like watching the news in the morning, do sit ups or walk on a treadmill at the same time. Time goes by fast when your mind is distracted.

SYSTEMS FOR DE-STRESSIFICATION

WHEN HANDED LEMONS, MAKE LEMONADE OR JUGGLE

Learn to leverage your psychology to diffuse your stress levels.

Your psychology is your state of mind throughout your day. It's what tells you when you wake up whether you are in a good mood and what creates stress when you encounter obstacles.

Treat it like a wild horse that you have come to tame. The wild horse is running outside your dude ranch, and it is your job to get it inside the corral and harness it. Once you get it inside your corral, take it where you want to go. If the horse gets mad and throws you off, it is your job to get back on and ride it.

Your mind is often like the wild horse, and more often than not, it is outside the corral, not in your control. Stress is like the horse kicking you off, leaving you on the ground of despair.

You can teach your mind to obey your intention. Let's look at an example. You hit traffic on the way to work that will make you late. You can start screaming at the cars and hit the steering wheel with your fist, all of which create stress, or you can call the office, alert your assistant, turn on the radio, search the stations until you find something you love, and rock on until you reach your office.

In the first scenario, you are a victim of your wild horse; in the second, you are in control with the "reins" of thought navigation firmly in your hands.

Learn to focus on solutions and outcomes, not problems, and you will begin to diffuse your anxiety and stress levels. When you focus only on a problem(s), it or they take on a life of their own, and magnify just by giving it attention. When you focus on results, your mind will spin into creative problem solving mode, keeping your laser intelligence tuned to the puzzle at hand. Next time you are stressed, focus on turning the problem inside out to create a remedy. Think: there are no problems, only challenges that require your creativity, ingenuity, and resolve.

Stress management is one of the most difficult but also one of the most essential HP habits to develop. It provides you with an important tool to redirect anger and frustration into acceptance and creativity. Resolving to find a positive action to replace one that is stressed is not easy; it takes practice.

FIX IT, ACCEPT IT, OR FORGET IT

Here are three guidelines for dealing with stress: fix it, accept it, or forget it.

If you can fix the problem, try several solutions until you find one that works. Finding a solution to a difficult problem is more productive and positive than fixating on what caused the problem. Your first line of stress management should always be to look at the remedies at your disposal.

If you can fix the problem but choose not to, accept whatever outcome it generates, and move on. Shift your focus to other issues that need your attention. Focusing on something you have decided not to address is a waste of valuable time.

If you can't fix the problem and it is completely out of your control, accept it. Redirect yourself toward something that takes your mind off the negative circumstances (music, talking to someone you know or love).

MOTIVATE, COMPENSATE, ELIMINATE, BALANCE, AND INTEGRATE

This strategy has served our clients over the years. Once you have developed systems for staying motivated (it may take more than three months of practice for new health habits to stick), break the old habits that no longer serve you. Compensating is the second-most important habit you can develop.

For example, if you want to eat something sweet every night at eleven p.m., what can you do? Find a replacement that is satisfying, such as a piece of fruit or a handful of nuts, for two weeks. After that, use the delay strategy: if you can delay the craving, reward yourself the next day, as long as it is eaten early in the day when your body is active, and not in the evenings, when your metabolism slows down and the body prepares for rest.

After you have learned to compensate, your next challenge is to eliminate. If you need to eliminate cigarettes, start with cutting back.. Keep trying until you beat it. Nicotine patches are helpful once you have kicked the habit. If not, cut back every day until you succeed This reinforces that you can do the impossible. When you are ready to "be the boss" of your health, end this habit with a vengeance. Cigarettes destroy your lungs and immune system, and they are a constant reminder that you are not in control of your life.

Your last two final steps are to balance and integrate. Once you have mastered motivation, substituted bad habits with good ones, and eliminated some of your weak link habits, you are ready to balance and integrate your new systems. You become the captain of your health "ship" and the "pilot" of your fate.

REMEMBER, YOU NEED TO PRACTICE HEALTH EVERY DAY TO BECOME GOOD AT IT.

Congratulations! You have taken the first steps in your journey to mastering high-performance physiology: educating yourself, increasing your awareness, and acquiring the "tools" for your superior health toolbox. Once you begin using the tools, you will look and feel better.

Life is full of challenges, and the better your health, the better you can cope with them. The better your brain works, the better you work.

Be unrelenting in your quest to improve your physiology. You will find untold rewards in achieving superior health: greater energy and productivity, more consistently elevated moods, and stronger motivation, to name a few.

Once you make a commitment to improve your health, you will see changes. Some come quickly, and others take time.

The key is to stay committed. Be resolute, and get back on track when you lose your footing. Everyone slips from time to time. Remember that learning something new—how to ride a bicycle, water ski, or give a motivational speech—does not happen with one try. You fall off the bike and have to pick yourself up, but you learn by getting back on the bike and trying again.

If you stick with your decision to become a high performer and execute your Action Plan, there is no limit to what you can accomplish.

Welcome to your new and improved high-performance physiology. You are entering an enriched phase of your life. Work it, and you will reap the rewards of superior health, productivity, and performance.

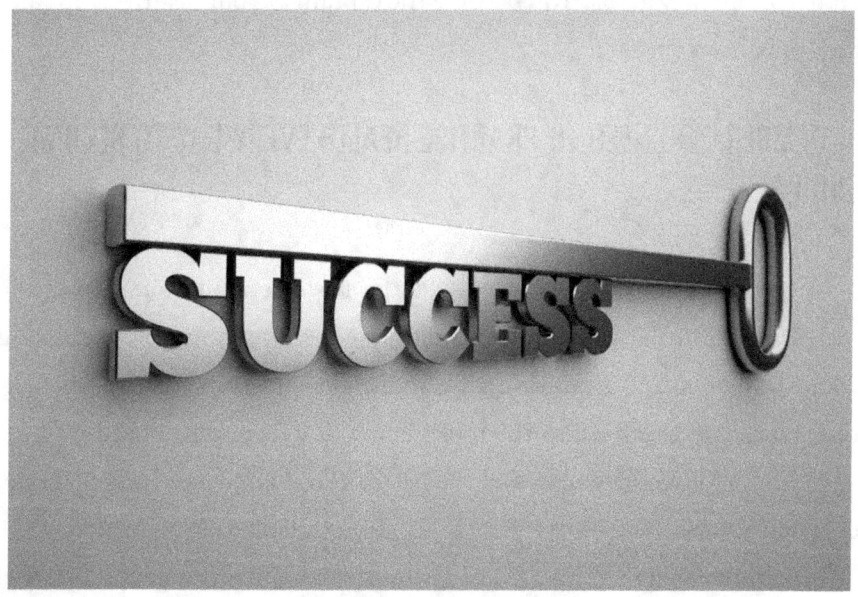

NOTES

✧ ✧ ✧

THE GOOD GUYS: FOODS HIGH IN NUTRIENTS

FOODS THAT BOOST YOUR IMMUNITY

Berries

Broccoli family vegetables

Carrots

Citrus Fruits

Dark Leafy Greens

Figs and Dates

Garlic

Flaxseed

Legumes (lentils, peas, beans, chick peas, mung beans)

Oats

Olives and olive oil

Pomegranate

Herbs and spices

FOODS THAT BOOST BRAIN POWER

Berries

Salmon

Organic or Omega 3 eggs

Spinach

Raw almonds

Bell peppers

Carrots

Avocado

Flax seed

Dark Chocolate

HIGH FUNCTIONAL FOODS

FRUITS: ORGANIC, FRESH

Apples

Berries (all kinds, blueberries, raspberries, strawberries)

Lemons and limes

Oranges

Bananas

Avocado

Grapes

Mango

Papaya

Kiwi

Grapefruits

Plums

Cherries

VEGETABLES: ORGANIC, FRESH

Dark leafy greens (arugula, **kale, spinach**, collards, turnip greens, swiss chard, romaine lettuce)

Artichokes

Bell peppers (red, orange, green)

Hot peppers (jalapeno, chile)

Dandelions

Onions

Tomato

Celery

Leeks

Zucchini

NUTS AND SEEDS

All kinds, preferably raw and organic:

Flax seeds

Chia seeds

Almonds

Cashews

Brazil nuts

Walnuts

Pine nuts

Hemp seeds

Macadamia

OILS

Cold-pressed, extra virgin olive oil
Raw, cold-pressed virgin coconut oil
Chia

WHOLE GRAINS

Quinoa
Oats
Millet
Buckwheat
Rye

HERBS AND SPICES

Garlic
Ginger
Cayenne pepper
Apple Vinegar cold pressed
Raw Chocolate
Cumin
Curries
Turmeric
Cinnamon
Dill

SUGAR SUBSTITUTES

Raw honey

Stevia

Date sugar

Agave syrup

Coconut nectar

MISCELLANEOUS

Organic eggs

Raw (non homogenized) milk, yoghurt and cheese

Fish

Raw protein powder

Green powder (spirulina, wheat grass, blue green algae, chlorella)

Fermented vegetables (kim chee, sauerkraut)

THE BAD GUYS: FOODS TO AVOID

- **Foods in packages** that are highly processed; these are "dead" foods that lack high quality nutrients. Most of the food you buy in a package should come from an organic food supplier who usually screens products for quality;
- **Soda**: high levels of empty nutrients and/or harmful sugar substitutes and high fructose corn syrup;
- **Deep fried foods**: If cooked in oils which are highly heated, it produces acrylamide, a known carcinogen (think donuts, French fries);
- **Canned foods**: the metal containers, high salt content, and preservatives are harmful;
- **Cereals, baked goods, bread** (small amounts of whole grain breads is okay);
- **Desserts, jams, candy**, and all items on the grocery shelves with high sugar content;
- **Fast food** masquerading as food;
- **Cold cuts** of meat are full of additives and preservatives, like sodium nitrate. It mixes with natural juices in meats and can lead to the development of carcinogens;
- **Milk and butter products**: they're not made today in ways which provide your body with health benefits. Find some alternatives in your favourite organic store (rice milk, almond milk, walnut butter, olive butter);

- Margarine
- Non-dairy creamer
- **Five ingredients** you should avoid:
    a. **High Fructose Corn syrup**
    b. **Artificial Sweeteners**, like amino Sweet, NutraSweet, Equal
    c. **MSG** (monosodium glutamate)
    d. **Sodium nitrate** (in cold cut meats, like salami, bologna and corned beef, bacon, hot dogs, and ham)
    e. **Trans fat**

FOODS YOU WANT TO MINIMIZE:

- Sugar and Sweets,
- Juice , unless homemade
- Gourmet coffee drinks
- Alcohol
- Most bottled salad dressings

A CLEANSING (FASTING) PLAN TO ASSIST YOUR NATURAL DETOXIFICATION

Before you attempt a serious assisted detoxification therapy, you must first understand that it is a process which enhances the body's own detoxification mechanism. Its purpose is to eliminate toxins that have accumulated in your body and brain, particularly in fat tissue.

Detoxification is the body's mechanism for protecting you from harmful substances that can damage your internal organs. The body has an innate internal intelligence to identify and remove toxins; however, if they cannot be removed safely (the toxic burden problem), they must be stored in a place that does the least harm to you (hence the reason adipose tissue is the preferred storage site for toxic debris). This is not to say that this is the only place toxins are stored; toxins can accumulate anywhere in the body and in the brain.

We point this out because it is important to recognize that if you have never cleansed via detoxification before, you may experience some unpleasant symptoms as the toxins are released into your blood stream. Keep in mind that this is normal; the body can find various ways to remove toxins, through the skin, blood, urine, etc. As a result, you may have symptoms like tiredness, skin irritations, bad breath, headaches, or nausea. This usually occurs during the first few days, but it can also occur at any time. This is not unusual; it is part of the process.

In addition, some people can experience a healing "crisis," which is when the body eliminates a strong toxic accumulation; this can result in a brief, but sometimes intense episode of feeling unwell as the body cleanses.

Having said this, we recommend that our readers find a qualified practitioner in Functional Medicine to guide them in an Assisted Detoxification Therapy. If this is not possible, we have provided you with an easy to follow cleansing plan: simple steps you can take to assist the body's internal detoxification.

CLEANSING (FASTING) PLAN:

Set aside TWO WEEKS where you can focus on cleansing: One week to prepare your mind and body, the second week for fasting from processed foods, caffeine, foods high in sugar and additives, and breads, pastas, dairy, meats and heavy oils.

For cleansing purposes, it is important that we not only increase the kinds of foods that are rich in nutrients, but we must also reduce the foods that burden our internal detoxification machinery, like the ones mentioned above and throughout this book. Doing this will maximize the supply of nutrients to the brain and organs and optimize the pathways for detoxification.

WEEK ONE: PREPARE YOUR MIND AND BODY

1. **Think about what you are trying to accomplish**: removing some of the harmful toxins that you have accumulated in your body from diet and lifestyle. To start, first identify what factors are potentially the main contributors to toxic accumulation.

2. **Reduce your exposure to toxins**. Focus on your lifestyle first, and reduce the following toxins as much as possible in the prep week: alcohol, coffee, cigarettes, fast foods, fried foods, packaged foods, saturated and trans fats. You should also reduce your meat consumption drastically; try and go vegetarian for a week leading up to fasting. Also, if you can reduce caffeinated beverages like coffee or switch to green tea (both have caffeine, but tea has less), this is highly recommended. Coffee can be a serious addiction and creates many toxins; removing it early on will make your second week of fasting that much easier.

    Other, not so obvious toxins are chemicals in body care products, household cleansers, and air pollution. Try and avoid these products too, or begin substituting "greener" products.

3. **Increase your consumption of water**: this is one of the essential pieces of assisting natural detoxification. Think of flushing out the debris that has accumulated in your body over the years and decades. You need water, and lots of it, to get the flow of nutrients and waste into and out of your cells.

    Don't make excuses; figure out a strategy for getting your pure, unadulterated water intake up to 10-12 glasses a day. If you don't have filtered water, locate a store which sells a simple device for purifying water (for example, Brita).

4. **Start exercising**. This, like water, is essential to helping the body eliminate toxins. If you do not have a regular exercise routine, then start walking. Set aside at least 30-45 minutes

every day for a walk out in the fresh air, or a jog on a treadmill (you know where they are, find a gym and get weekly passes. Better still, join one).

5.   **Increase your consumption of fresh fruits and vegetables drastically, and prepare your mind and refrigerator** for Week Two. Remember what you are trying to accomplish: it is only two weeks of your life; it is manageable if you have the right mind set.

IF YOU CAN MANAGE THESE FIVE STEPS, YOU WILL HAVE ALREADY BEGUN TO CLEANSE INTERNALLY.

WEEK TWO: FASTING IN THREE PARTS

PART ONE "Step down" (first three days of second week)

1.   You are now preparing for fasting (Day One, Two, and Three of Week Two). The foods we suggest you reduce in Week One (mentioned at the onset), are now eliminated. Think of it as giving your digestive system a small vacation from processed foods, foods that are hard to digest, fried foods, meats, caffeine, foods high in sugar and additives, as well as breads, pastas, dairy, and heavy oils. If some of you have fasted for religious purposes, you may recognize a similar regimen.

241

2. Avoid alcohol, cigarettes and recreational drugs. Absolutely no junk food or fast food, and no caffeinated products, which over-stimulate the liver. If you find it impossible to cut nicotine, cut back as much as possible.

3. Avoid foods that irritate your stomach because they are hard to digest. This group of food includes wheat and dairy products, and fried foods. Switch to brown rice, quinoa (a South American rice-like grain) and millet.

4. Try and say "No!" to sugar products completely for the entire week; they deplete your minerals and interfere with your ability to control your blood sugar.

5. Eliminate meats completely; we are giving your digestive tract a break from foods hard to digest. Meats are eliminated while cleansing because they are high in protein, saturated fats and produce acidity. They also may contain hormones and antibiotics which are difficult for our livers to detoxify. Remember, we are trying to enhance the body's ability to remove toxins. Avoid those foods with a high content of toxins.

6. Increase your alkalinity by radically increasing consumption of vegetables. Vegetables are Nature's Way of keeping us more alkaline; and therefore healthier. An acidic diet uses up many of our important minerals. Meat, hard cheeses, sugar, alcohol, and too many grain products, like breads and pasta, are all acidic. Particularly helpful are vegetables like beets, broccoli, cauliflower, cabbage, brussel sprouts, and kale.)

PART TWO: (Two) days of FASTING (Day 4 & 5,)

7.   After your three days of "Step down," you will have two days of fasting with fruits and vegetables. Ideally, this should be done with a juicer and blender in order to provide you with the freshest and most vitamin/micronutrient enriched fasting drink. However, if you do not have this equipment at home, or do not live in a city where you might find a store that offers this service (organic markets, health food stores, and even gyms now have juice bars), then find a local neighborhood store that sells high quality juices.

Our recommended routine is to start each morning with 2 glasses of water, followed by a fruit mixer, using any fruits except orange and grapefruit.

For lunch, try to juice vegetables. Root vegetables are particularly cleansing, like carrots and beets.

For Dinner, enjoy vegetable soups and broths.

Herbal teas and bouillion vegetable broths are acceptable as in between snacks during this time also.

If you need ideas for drinks, try using Google; the internet is full of websites devoted to drinks for fasting. Just remember that you should be strict: no dairy, like yoghurt, milk etc. Below are some suggested websites for smoothies and drinks:

http://www.fitnessblender.com/v/article-detail/Fruit-and-Vegetable-Juice-Recipes-for-Fasting-Detox-Juice-Recipes/am/

http://www.incrediblesmoothies.com/juice-fasting/
my-5-day-green-juice-fast-experience/

8. Last but not least: DRINK LOTS AND LOTS OF WATER

PART 3: STEP UP (last two days)

1. Return to the eating routines of the first three days: keep meat out of your diet, and replace with high quality vegetable protein sources like beans, lentils, vegetables stir fry over brown rice and quinoa, etc.

2. Keep drinking the high quality vegetable and fruit juices

3. Keep drinking lots of water to keep the "flush" going.

REFERENCES

[1] Daniel Amen Lecture. "Creating A High Performance Brain," *Summer Institute for Sport,* 2012, May 2012 http://www.summerinstituteforsport.com/resources/psychology-and-motivation/psychology-and-motivation-videos/dr-amencreating-a-high-performance

[2] Felicia Kliment, *The Acid Alkaline Balance Diet.* New York: McGraw-Hill, 2002, Chapter 1.

[3] Sidney MacDonald Baker. *Detoxification and Healing.* New York: McGraw Hill, 2008, 14.

[4] Patrick Holford. *Optimal Nutrition for the Mind.* North Bergen, NJ; Basic Health Publications, Inc., 4.

[5] Holford, 5.

[6] Baker, 14.

[7] Patricia Fitzgerald, *The Detox Solution.* Santa Monica, CA, Illumination Press, 2001, 4.

[8] Natasha Campbell-McBride. *Gut and Psychology Syndrome. GAPS-What is it?* retrieved from http://www.gaps.me/preview/?page_id=20.

[9] HOPES: Huntington's Outreach Project for Education, at Stanford. Brain-derived neurotrophic factor (BDNF), June 26,2010, retrieved from https://www.stanford.edu/group/hopes/cgi-bin/wordpress/2010/06/brain-derived-neurotrophic-factor-bdnf/#can-ex

[10] Dr. Mark Hyman, "Is there Toxic Waste In Your Body," May 19, 2010, http://drhyman.com/blog/2010/05/19/is-there-toxic-waste-in-your-body-2/

[11] World Health Organization World, Constitution of WHO, retreived from http://www.who.int/en. http://www.who.int/governance/eb/who_constitution_en.pdf

[12] Fitzgerald, 8.

[13] Symeon Rodger, Rock Solid Health Qi Gong Manual and Videos. *Rock Solid Life Systems, Inc.* 2010. retrieved from http://taichiforseniors.net/unity-of-mind-and-body.

[14] Fitzgerald, 10.

[15] Holford, 5.

[16] Fitzgerald, 15, 32.

[17] David Servan Schreiber. *Anti Cancer A New Way of Life* New York, NY: Viking Penguin, 2008, 132.

[18] Holford, 1.

[19] Patrick Holford and G. Roberts. 'Effect of vitamin and mineral supplementation on intelligence of school children," *Lancet*, Vol. 2 (8578), 1998, 140–3.

[20] Yvonne Wettergren, "Guts, germs and genes! Who is ruling whom?" The Sahlggrenska Academy at Gothenburg, retrieved from **probiotics. se**

[21] *Nutrition in Clinical Practice* 2012 Apr;27(2):201-14

[22] Lennart Cedgård, MD, GM Wasa Medicals, Gothenburg Anna Widell BSc in Bioscience, Wasa Medicals, Gothenburg. "The intestinal microflora, the immune system and probiotics." *Swedish Medical Journal*, 50-2001 retrieved from **probiotics.se**

[23] "Why Probiotics". retrieved from **http://morgellonsfocusonhealth. com/probiotics**

[24] Yvonne Wettergren. Guts, germs and genes! Who is ruling whom?

[25] Health Benefits of Taking Probiotics. *Harvard Medical School: Family Guide* retrieved from http://www.health.harvard.edu/fhg/updates/ update0905c.shtml.

[26] Natasha Campbell-McBride. *Gut and Psychology Syndrome.*

[27] Dr. Mercola interviews Dr McBride-Campbell. Dr. Mercola Interviews Dr. Natasha Campbell-McBride about Immunity and Gut Flora.

[28] Daniel Amen, "Creating a High-Performance Brain," *The Summer Institute for Sport,* lecture. http://www.summerinstituteforsport.com/resources/psychology-and-motivation/psychology-and-motivation-videos/dr-amencreating-a-high-performance.

[29] Holford. 4.

[30] Holford. 13.

[31] Holford. 23.

[32] D.O Rudin. "The major psychoses and neuroses as omega-3 essential fatty acid deficiency syndrome substrate pellagra," *Biol Psychiatry.* Vol. 16(9), 1981, 837-50.

[33] Holford. 38-40.

[34] Holford. 40.

[35] Holford. 37.

[36] Council for Responsible Nutrition's 20th anniversary annual conference in Washington, D.C. 1993

[37] Michael McGinnes, ND Ernst. *Preventive nutrition: a historic perspective and future economic outlook.* In: Bendich A, Deckelbaum FJ, Editors. Primary and Secondary Preventive Nutrition. Humana Press, Totowa, NJ, 2001

[38] Dr Fuhrman. How to Live Your Life, 2004-2012, **retrieved from** http://www.drfuhrman.com/library/are-you-a-nutritarian.aspx

[39] Men's Journal. "Maximize Your Micronutrients". April 28, 2011. retrieved from **http://archive.mensjournal.com/andiscores.**

[40] Holford, 46-51.

[41] Live Strong: The Limitless Potential of You, What is the Recommended Daily Intake of Fat Grams, 2012, **retrieved from** http://www.livestrong.com/article/47612-recommended-daily-intake-fat-grams/#ixzz2AbDjO43Z.

[42] High Sugar Consumption: MIT Researchers. *MIT Conference Proceedings on Research Strategies for Assessing the Behavioral Effects of Foods and Nutrients*, 1982.

[43] A. G. Schauss. "Nutrition and Behavior: Complex Interdisciplinary Research", *Nutrition and Health*, 3:9-37, 1984. A.G. Schauss, "Nutrition and Behavior," *Journal of Applied Nutrition*, Vol 35(1), 1983, 30-35.

[44] Tuula E. Tuormaa "The Adverse Effects of Food Additives on Health: A review of the Literature with special Emphasis on Childhood Hyperactivity." *Journal of Orthomolecular Medicine* Vol 9,Nov 4,1994. P225 retrieved from http://www.orthomolecular.org/library/jom/1994/pdf/1994-v09n04-p225.pdf.

[45] Holford. 61–62.

[46] Kliment, 5.

[47] Roger J. Williams. *Nutrition Against Disease.* New York, NY: Bantam Books. http://americannutritionassociation.org/newsletter/nutrition-against-disease-roger-j-williams-phd.

[48] F. Batmanghelid, MD, *Your Body's Many Cries for Water.* Global Health Solutions, Inc. 1-10.

[49] Batmanghelid, 3.

[50] Batmanghelid, 17.

[51] Batmanghelid, 17.

[52] Albert Grazia. "Dangers of Chronic Dehydration," *Nutrition, Herbs, and Natural Healing for Health and Wellness,* February 2012 retrieved from http://nutritioninfo.tripod.com/id19.html

[53] Ibid.

[54] Christopher MaGovern, *ABC News,* February 14, 2012.

[55] Daniel P. Reid. *The Tao of Health, Sex and Longevity.* CITY: Simon and Schuster, 1989, 156.

[56] Reid, *Tao of Detox.* Healing Art Press, 2006, 81.

[57] BBC News. "No Sleep Means No New Brain Cells." *BBC News.* February 10, 2007 retrieved from www.news.bbc.co.uk/2/hi/6347043.stm.

[58] Ibid.

[59] Dr. Damien Léger, *Archives Internal Medicine,* September 2006.

[60] Phyliss C. Zee, MD, Fred W. Turek, PhD. *Archives of Internal Medicine,* September 18, 2006, 166(16). 1686-1688.

[61] Sleep Disorders and Sleep Deprivation: An Unmet Health Problem. Report, 2006 Institute of Medicine of the National Academies. http://www.iom.edu/~/media/Files/Report%20Files/2006/Sleep-Disorders-and-Sleep-Deprivation-An-Unmet-Public-Health-Problem/ Sleepforweb.pdf

[62] http://www.medicineonline.com/news/12/6175/Nasal-allergies-significantly-impact-sleep-quality.html.

[63] Baker, 148–9.

[64] Theodore Baroody. "Sunlight", *Alkalize or Die.* City, CA: EcclecticPublishing, 1991, 65.

[65] Dr Joseph Mercola, . "Vitamin D Deficiency and Disease," *Dark Deceptions*. Nashville, Tennessee; Thomas Nelson Publishers, 2008. 66.

[66] WEB, MD. "Vitamin D" retrieved from http://www.webmd.com/diet/ vitamin-d-deficiency?page=2.

[67] Daniel Goleman, *The New York Times: Science.* "Relaxation: Surprising Benefits Detected. May 13,1986. http://www.nytimes.com/1986/05/13/ science/relaxation-surprising-benefits-detected.html?pagewanted=all.

[68] Herbert Benson. "Relaxation," *Health Insights Today*, 69.

[69] Daniel Redwood interview with Herbert Benson, *Health Insights Today*. Fall 2008, Volume 1, Issue 3, p 1-5. retrieved from http://www.healthinsightstoday.com/articles/v1i3/pdrelaxation_response_benson.pdf

[70] Tracy Roizman. Livestrong.com: The Limitless Potential of You. "The Purpose of EPA, DHA, and GLA". Feb. 6,2011. retrieved from http://www.livestrong.com/article/375290-the-purpose-of-epa-dha-gla/#ixzz2J9z3PRsd.

[71] Holford, 27.

[72] Quest for Health Library. Evening Primrose oil. retrieved from http://www.questhealthlibrary.com/other-supplements/evening-primrose-oil.

[73] Prevention. retrieved from http://www.prevention.com/superspices/index.html. 7 Superspices. Paige Nestel. 2012.

[74] David Servan-Schreiber. *Anti Cancer A New Way of Life*. New York: Viking Penguin, 2008, 60-63.

[75] Gary D. Stoner, Ph.D. "Berries and Cancer", *Medical College of Wisconssin*. retrieved from http://berryhealth.org/presentations/Cancer-Stoner.pdf

[76] Sara Morse, "Pomegranate Health Benefits," Suite 101. 1997. Pomegranate Health Benefits. | retrieved from Suite101.com

http://suite101.com/article/pomegranate-health-benefits-a222888#ixzz1w5vxVQMW.

[77] Anne Copley, *Challenging Behavior.* U.K.; Network Continuum, 2006. 1-8.

[78] Copley, 1, 10, 11.

[79] Copley, 2.

[80] Kevin Rail. "List of Complex Carbohydrate Foods." Dec. 7, 2011. Livestrong-The Limitless Potential of You. 2012. retrieved from http://www.livestrong.com/article/27398-list-complex-carbohydrates-foods/#ixzz1rBuq4y3F.

[81] Lawrence Girard. "Definition of Simple Sugars." eHOW 2012 retrieved from http://www.ehow.com/about_6553812_definition-simple-sugars.html.

[82] Ibid.

[83] Mercola.com. Avoid This Food to Help Slow Aging. Dr. Mercola. 2012. retrieved from http://articles.mercola.com/sites/articles/archive/2012/02/22/how-sugar-accelerates-aging.aspx.

[84] Patrick Holford, *Optimal Nutrition for the Mind.* North Bergen, NJ; Basic Health Publications, Inc., 58.

[85] Amen Clinic.2012. retrieved from http://www.amenclinics.net.

[86] Erik Odom. "List of Foods with the Highest Amount of Monounsaturated Fat." Dec. 20, 2011. Livestrong-The Limitless Potential

of You, 2012. retrieved from http://www.livestrong.com/article/30663-list-foods-highest-amount-monounsaturated/#ixzz1wLuOogc7.

[87] Daniel Amen. *Use Your Brain to Change Your Age.* New York: Crown Archetype, 2012, 124, www.crownpublishing.com.

[88] Paul Pitchford. *Healing With Whole Foods.* Berkley, CA: North Atlantic Books, 2002. 123.

[89] J. Yiamouyiannis. *Fluoride: The Aging Factor.* Delaware, OH: Health Action Press, 1986, 43-69.

[90] Anna L. Choi, Guifan Sun, Ying Zhang, and Philippe Grandjean . *Developmental Fluoride Neurotoxicity: A Systematic Review and Meta-Analysis* retrieved from http://www.ncbi.nlm.nih.gov/pmc/articles/PMC3491930/pdf/ehp.1104912.pdf

[91] Yiamouyiannis, *Fluoride: The Aging Factor.* 43-69.

[92] Pitchford, 124.

[93] Martin Riny. "Which Alkaline Ionized Water Benefits Should You Consider." March 22,2012. *Ionized Water FAQS*, 2012. retrieved from http://www.ionizedwaterfaq.com/alkaline-ionized-water-benefits-health.

[94] Gretchen Reynolds. "How Exercise Can Lead to a Better Brain," April 18, 2012, *New York Times.* retrieved from http://www.nytimes.com/2012/04/22/magazine/how-exercise-could-lead-to-a-better-brain.html?pagewanted=all.

[95] Juliet Harpe. "Three Good Exercises For the Circulatory System." July 12, 2011. Livestrong – The Limitless Potential of You, 2012. retrieved from http://www.livestrong.com/article/491021-three-good-exercises-for-the-circulatory-system/#ixzz29utd6q2D.

[96] C. M. Friedenreich and M. R. Orenstein. "Physical Acitvity and Cancer Prevention: Etiologic Evidence and Biological Mechanisms," *Journal of Nutrition* 132, no. 11, supp. (2002): 34565–645.

[97] Daniel Amen. *Use Your Brain to Change Your Age.* New York: Crown Archetype, 2012, 124. www.crownpublishing.com.

[98] Amen, 125-130.

[99] Grethchen Reynolds. "PhysEd: How Exercising Keeps Your Cells Young." *New York Times*, January 27, 2010, 12:01 a.m., retrieved from http://well.blogs.nytimes.com/2010/01/27/phys-ed-how-exercising-keeps-your-cells-young.

[100] "Lowering Physical Activity Impairs Glycemic Control in Healthy Volunteers" study published in *Medicine and Science Sports and Exercise*, February 2012. retrieved from http://www.ncbi.nlm.nih.gov/pubmed/21716152 http://munews.missouri.edu/news-releases/2011/0823-mu-study-links-inactivity-with-risk-factors-for-type-2-diabetes.

[101] Anne Marie W.Petersen and Bente Klarlund Pedersen. "The Anti-Inflammatory Effect of Exercise" article published in the *Journal of Applied Physiology*, April 1, 2005, vol. 98, no. 41154-1162 retrieved from http://jap.physiology.org/content/98/4/1154.full#content-block.

[102] 'Exercise to Improve Your Body and Your Brain" Peak Fitness presented by Mercola.com. retrieved from http://fitness.mercola.com/sites/fitness/exercises.aspx.

[103] Servan-Schreiber, 187.

[104] National Institute for Clinical Excellence, Depression: The Management of Depression in Primary and Secondary Care, *NICE Guideline Second Draft Consultation,* London 2003.

[105] Grethchen Reynolds, " How Exercise Could Lead to a Better Brain." *New York Times*, April 18, 2012. retrieved from http://www.nytimes.com/2012/04/22/magazine/how-exercise-could-lead-to-a-better-brain.html?pagewanted=all&_r=0.

[106] Media release "Preventing dementia: new research by VCH and UBC shows trajectory of cognitive decline can be altered in seniors at risk for dementia," April 23, 2012, *Archives of Internal Medicine,* retrieved from http://www.publicaffairs.ubc.ca/2012/04/23/preventing-dementia-new-research-by-vch-and-ubc-shows-the-trajectory-of-cognitive-decline-can-be-altered-in-seniors-at-risk-for-dementia.

[107] Gretchen Reynolds, "How Exercise Benefits the Brain." *New York Times*, November 30, 2011, retrieved from http://well.blogs.nytimes.com/2011/11/30/how-exercise-benefits-the-brain

[108] M. Millan Sanchez, D. Das, J. L. Taylor, A. Noda, J. A. Yesavage, and A. Salehi. "BDNF polymorphism predicts the rate of decline in skilled task performance and hippocampal volume in healthy individual"

Translational Psychiatry Journal, October 25, 2011 retrieved from http://www.nature.com/tp/journal/v1/n10/full/tp201147a.html#aff1

[109] Gretchen Reynolds, "Why It's So Important to Keep Moving." *New York Times*, February 29, 2012. retrieved from http://well.blogs.nytimes.com/2012/02/29/why-its-so-important-to-keep-moving.

[110] Len Saputo and Nancy Faass, eds. *Boosting Immunity: Creating Wellness Naturally* Novato, CA: New Work Library, 2002, 112.

[111] Servan-Schreiber, 61-65.

[112] Peter M. Crosta. "Researchers Verify Link Between Type 2 Diabetes And Diet." *Medical News Today*, July 30, 2008. http://www.medicalnewstoday.com/articles/116513.php.

[113] Derived from the Alexis Carrel Papers, Special Collections Division, Georgetown University Library, Washington, DC.

[114] Kliment. *The Acid Alkaline Balance Diet.* New York: McGraw-Hill, 2002, xi.

[115] Kliment, 8.

[116] Pitchford, 274-279.

[117] Holford, 4.

[118] http://www.drweil.com/drw/u/QAA400149/balancing-omega-3-and-omega-6.html

[119] Janice K. Kiecolt-Glaser, Ph.D., Martha A. Belury, Ph.D., Kyle Porter, M.A.S., David Beversdorf, M.D.,Stanley Lemeshow, Ph.D., and Ronald Glaser, Ph.D. Depressive Symptoms, n-6:n-3 Fatty Acids, and Inflammation in Older Adults Janice K. Kiecolt-Glaser. *US National Library of Medicine, National Institutes of Health Psychomsom.* Med. 2007 Apr 69(3). 217-24. Epub March 2007. retrieved from http://www.ncbi.nlm.nih.gov/pmc/articles/PMC2856352/

[120] US National Library of Medicine, National Institutes of Health Psychomsom. Med. 2007 Apr 69(3). 217-24. Epub March 2007 http://www.ncbi.nlm.nih.gov/pmc/articles/PMC2856352/

[121] Janice K. Kiecolt-Glaser, Ph.D, Depressive Symptoms, n-6:n-3 Fatty Acids, and Inflammation in Older Adults.

[122] Elizabeth Scott "Stress: How It Affects Your Body, and How You Can Stay Healthier." About.com/Guide, updated May 14, 2011 retrieved from http://stress.about.com/od/stresshealth/a/stresshealth.html.

[123] Sue Shellenbarger, "When Stress Is Good for You." *Wall Street Journal*: Europe Edition, January 24, 2012, retrieved from http://online.wsj.com/article/SB10001424052970204301404577171192704005250.html.

[124] Scott, retrieved from http://stress.about.com/od/stresshealth/a/stresshealth.html.

[125] Theodore F. Robles, Ronald Glaser, and Janice K. Kiecolt Glaser, "Out of Balance: A New Look at Chronic Stress, Depression and Immunity." retrieved from http://uppitysciencechick.homestead.com/robles_stress_dep_immune.pdf

[126] Stress and Coping Mechanisms adapted from Mayo Clinic, retrieved from http://www.mayoclinic.com/health/stress-management/SR00032 http://www.mayoclinic.com/health/stress-management/SR00032/ NSECTIONGROUP=2 http://www.mayoclinic.com/health/stress/ SR00001.

[127] Baker, p. xvi- xviii.

[128] H.E.A.L. Medical Corp, 2000 Van Ness, Suite 501A, San Francisco 94109, http://marshanunleymd.com/

[129] Dr. Mark Hyman, "Is There Toxic Waste in Your Body?" May 19,2010, retrieved from http://drhyman.com/blog/2010/05/19/ is-there-toxic-waste-in-your-body-2/

[130] High Fructose Corn Syrup Linked to Liver Scarring, Research Suggests." *Science Daily*, 118. www.sciencedaily.com/releases/ 2010/03/100322204628

[131] Carolyn Guilford. "High Fructose Corn Syrup", *The Savannah Tribune*, September 24, 2008 retrieved from http://www.savannahtribune.com/ news/2008-09-24/health/015.html.

[132] Acute Exposure Guidelines Levels for Selected Airborne Chemicals. Volume 4, *Subcommittee on Acute Exposure Guideline Levels Committee on Toxicology Board on Environmental Studies and Toxicology.* retrieved from **http://www.epa.gov/katrina/outreach/psa.html.**

[133] Chemical Hazard Data Availability Study, http://www.epa.gov/hpv/ pubs/general/hazchem.pdf.

[134] U.S. Department of Labor, Occupational Safety and Health Administration, 200 Constitution Ave., NW, Washington, DC, 20210. http://www.osha.gov/SLTC/hazardoustoxicsubstances/

[135] Chemical Hazard Data Availability Study http://www.epa.gov/hpv/pubs/general/hazchem.pdf

[136] Registration, Evaluation, Authorisation and Restriction of Chemicals (REACH) http://www.spring.gov.sg/Resources/Documents/Guidebook_Complying_with_REACH.pdf

[137] http://www.takepart.com/article/2012/09/11/your-cleaner-green-environmental-working-group-releases-cleaning-guide

[138] Ibid.

[139] World Resources Institute, 10 G Street NE Suite 800, Washington, DC 20002, USA http://www.wri.org/publication/content/8327

[140] U.S. Environmental Protection Agency, "Household Cleaners"(:60 secs, 941kb, MP3, **http://www.epa.gov/katrina/outreach/psa.html**

[141] "In Harm's Way", a study by The Clean Water Fund and Physicians for Social Responsibility, May 11, 2000.

[142] American Cancer Society. Cancer Facts and Figures. 2006. Special Section: Environmental Pollutants and Cancer" p.22, Atlanta, GA. http://www.cancer.org/acs/groups/content/@nho/documents/document/caff2006pwsecuredpdf.pdf.

[143] J. Onstot, R. Ayling, J. Stanley, Characterization of HRGC/MS Unidentified Peaks from *Analysis of Human Adipose Tissue*. Volume: Technical Approach. Washington, DC: U.S. Environmental Protection Agency Office of Toxic Substances (560/6-87-002a), 1987.

[144] Mercola.com http://articles.mercola.com/sites/articles/archive/2009/12/31/232-Toxic-Chemicals-found-in-10-Babies.aspx, December 31, 2009.

[145] J. Onstot, et al.

[146] "Is Your House Toxic?" Partners for Natural Health http://thepartnersfornaturalhealth.com/environmental-toxins-your-health.

[147] Rhonda Donahue, *The Pollution Inside You: What Is Your Body Dying to Say?* (Sheffield MA: Safe Goods, 2009).

[148] D. Eoin D, "Greenpeace Research Reveals Toxic Chemicals in Biggest Clothing Brands," retrieved from http://www.greenpeace.org.uk/blog/toxics/adidas-needs-earn-its-stripes-championing-toxic-free-future-20110823.

[149] Dr. Joseph Mercola. "Never Put This on Your Face or Skin", retrieved from http://www.mercolahealthyskin.com.

[150] David Jonasson, *Stockholm News*, December 17, 2012 http://www.stockholmnews.com/more.aspx?NID=8410.

[151] Neal, D.T., et al., "How do habits guide behavior? Perceived and actual triggers of habits in daily life" ; *Journal of Experimental Social Psychology* (2011), doi:10.1016/j.jesp.2011.10.011

[152] http://newsinhealth.nih.gov/issue/jan2012/feature1

[153] January 2012 *NIH Newsletter.* http://newsinhealth.nih.gov/issue/jan2012/feature